How to stop smoking during pregnancy and protect your baby: A definitive guide for pregnant women

Chandan Reddy Allam

Table of Contents

Introduction

Have you ever watched a caterpillar transform into a beautiful butterfly? It's a mesmerizing sight, isn't it? The way it sheds its old self, emerging with wings that carry it to new heights. Now, imagine you are that butterfly, ready to embark on the most extraordinary journey of your life - pregnancy. But here's the twist: you're also a passionate smoker. As the shock settles in, you realize that something needs to change. You have a tiny life growing inside you, relying on your every decision. Quitting smoking is a daunting task, but fear not, for within the pages of this book lies a definitive guide to help you stop smoking during pregnancy and protect your beautiful butterfly baby.

As I sat down to write this book, I couldn't help but become enraptured by the sheer importance of the topic at hand. Pregnancy, a time filled with anticipation, joy, and perhaps a touch of anxiety, is also a period where a mother's choices have a profound impact on the life, she carries within her. Smoking, that seemingly innocent habit you once indulged in, now takes on a whole new level of significance. It's time to extinguish the smoke, banish the ashes, and embrace a healthier future for both you and your precious baby.

This guide is not a mere collection of dos and don'ts. No, my dear reader, this is a love letter to every mother out there who finds herself at this crossroad. A road lined with temptations and uncertainties, where one wrong turn can steer you astray. But fear not, for within these pages, you will find the guiding light that will lead you towards a smoke-free life, one that nurtures and cherishes the little life blossoming within you.

Imagine a world where your baby is safe from the perils of smoking. Visualize the clean air filling your lungs and nourishing every cell of your body. Envision a future where your child's first breath is unpolluted, where their tiny lungs are free to explore the wonders of the world without the shackles of smoke. It's a beautiful image, isn't it? And let me tell you, my friend, that image can become a reality.

Taking inspiration from the delicate dance of a butterfly, we will explore the depths of the challenges you face and the strategies that will help you overcome them. Together, we will navigate the labyrinth of cravings, the withdrawal symptoms, and the emotional turmoil that accompanies this journey. But fear not, for I am here to hold your hand, to guide you through the darkness and into the radiant light of a smoke-free existence.

Through the perspective of a management consultant and author, I bring to you a unique perspective on understanding the risks associated with smoking during pregnancy. My experience in the healthcare industry has given me insight into the profound impact smoking can have on both mother and baby. I believe that every mother deserves the opportunity to make an informed decision, armed with knowledge and supported by practical advice.

In the pages that follow, I will not sugarcoat the difficulties you may encounter. Quitting smoking is a tumultuous path, but I promise you, my friend, it's a path worth taking. Together, we will explore the power of mindset, the strength of community, and the importance of self-care. We will uncover actionable tips and strategies that have been proven to help pregnant women successfully quit smoking, paving the way for a healthier future.

So, my dear reader, are you ready to embark on this transformative journey? To leave the cocoon of smoking behind and embrace the freedom of a smoke-free life? I invite you to turn the page, to delve into the chapters that await you, and to discover the inner strength that lies within. Together, we will conquer the challenges, surmount the cravings, and protect your beautiful butterfly baby. Let the metamorphosis begin!

Chapter 1: Understanding the Risks

The Impact of Smoking on Foetal Development

During pregnancy, a woman's body goes through numerous changes to support the growth and development of the baby. The placenta acts as a lifeline, providing the necessary nutrients, oxygen, and protection to the growing foetus. However, when a pregnant woman smokes, harmful substances like nicotine, carbon monoxide, and other chemicals are introduced into her body.

Nicotine, the addictive substance found in cigarettes, is particularly dangerous. When a pregnant woman smokes, nicotine rapidly enters her bloodstream and crosses the placenta, reaching the baby in a matter of seconds. This means that the developing foetus is exposed to the same level of nicotine as the mother, putting it at significant risk.

Once inside the foetus's body, nicotine disrupts the normal development process. It restricts the blood vessels, reducing blood flow and oxygen supply to the baby. This can lead to a condition called foetal hypoxia, where the baby is deprived of essential oxygen. Without enough oxygen, the baby's organs and tissues cannot develop properly. This can have serious consequences for the baby's overall growth and health.

The harmful chemicals in cigarette smoke also interfere with the baby's organ development. For example, smoking increases the risk of congenital heart defects, where the baby is born with structural abnormalities in the heart. The chemicals in cigarettes can damage the cells responsible for forming the heart valves and walls, leading to these defects. Additionally, smoking during pregnancy increases the risk of other birth defects, such as cleft lip and palate, limb abnormalities, and gastrointestinal problems.

Furthermore, smoking during pregnancy can impair the development of the baby's lungs. The chemicals in cigarette smoke can damage the delicate lung tissue, leading to reduced lung function and increased risk of respiratory problems later in life. Babies born to smoking mothers are more likely to develop asthma and other respiratory conditions, as their lungs haven't fully matured and are more susceptible to damage.

Another significant impact of smoking on foetal development is the increased risk of preterm birth. Smoking during pregnancy is a major risk factor for preterm labor, where the baby is born before 37 weeks of gestation. Premature babies are at a higher risk of numerous health complications, including respiratory distress syndrome, feeding difficulties, and developmental delays. They may require intensive medical care after birth and have a higher likelihood of experiencing long-term health issues.

Additionally, smoking during pregnancy increases the risk of low birth weight. Babies born to smoking mothers tend to weigh less than those born to non-smoking mothers. Low birth weight is associated with various health concerns, including increased risk of infections, developmental delays, and even mortality in severe cases. These babies may struggle to thrive and often require extra medical attention and support.

It is worth noting that the harmful effects of smoking during pregnancy can extend beyond birth. Studies have shown that children exposed to cigarette smoke in utero are more likely to face cognitive and behavioral issues. These children may have poorer attention spans, difficulties with learning and memory, and an increased risk of attention deficit hyperactivity disorder (ADHD).

The impact of smoking on foetal development is not limited to the mother's smoking habits alone. Second-hand smoke, the smoke breathed in by others in the vicinity, is equally harmful. Pregnant women who are exposed to second-hand smoke face similar risks to those who smoke themselves. The harmful chemicals in second-hand smoke can cross the placenta and harm the developing foetus just as easily as if the pregnant woman smoked directly.

Increased Risk of Miscarriage and Stillbirth

Miscarriage is a devastating event for any expectant mother. It is the sudden loss of a pregnancy before the 20th week. The emotional toll it takes on a woman is immeasurable, leaving her feeling empty and defeated. Unfortunately, smoking during pregnancy significantly increases the risk of experiencing a miscarriage.

Research has shown that smoking during pregnancy increases the risk of miscarriage by as much as 60%. The harmful chemicals present in cigarettes, such as nicotine, carbon monoxide, and various toxins, restrict the flow of oxygen and vital nutrients to the developing foetus. This deprivation of essential resources can lead to severe complications and ultimately result in the loss of the pregnancy.

Nicotine, in particular, is a highly addictive substance that constricts blood vessels and reduces blood flow. This constriction also restricts blood flow to the placenta, which is responsible for supplying oxygen and nutrients to the growing baby. Without a sufficient blood supply, the foetus may not develop properly and can lead to a miscarriage.

Furthermore, smoking increases the risk of a stillbirth, which is when the baby dies in the womb after the 20th week of pregnancy. The toxins in cigarettes not only affect the baby's development but can also damage the placenta, leading to complications that can be life-threatening for both the mother and the baby.

The emotional impact of experiencing a miscarriage or stillbirth due to smoking during pregnancy cannot be overstated. It is a heart-wrenching experience that leaves many women feeling guilt, shame, and a sense of failure. Society often places blame on the mother, further exacerbating these emotions.

The long-term effects of a miscarriage or stillbirth can also manifest physically. Studies have shown that women who have experienced a miscarriage or stillbirth are at a higher risk of developing mental health issues such as depression and anxiety. The grief and trauma associated with losing a pregnancy can have a profound impact on a woman's mental well-being.

In addition to the emotional and psychological effects, smoking during pregnancy can also have long-term physical consequences for the mother. Women who smoke during pregnancy are at an increased risk of developing complications such as ectopic pregnancy and placental abruption. Ectopic pregnancy occurs when the fertilized egg implants outside the uterus, usually in the fallopian tubes. This condition is life-threatening and requires immediate medical intervention.

Placental abruption, on the other hand, is when the placenta separates from the uterine wall before the baby is born. This can lead to heavy bleeding and deprive the baby of oxygen and nutrients. Both ectopic pregnancy and placental abruption are serious medical emergencies that can result in significant complications for both the mother and the baby.

Moreover, smoking during pregnancy can also lead to complications during childbirth. Women who smoke are more likely to have a premature birth, where the baby is born before 37 weeks of gestation. Premature babies are at a higher risk of developing health issues such as respiratory problems, developmental delays, and even long-term disabilities.

As a management consultant and author, I have witnessed the devastating effects of smoking during pregnancy on both the mother and the baby. The pain and anguish experienced by women who have lost a pregnancy due to smoking are heartbreaking. That is why I am passionate about spreading awareness and providing support for pregnant women who are struggling to quit smoking.

In the following chapters of this book, we will delve deeper into the strategies and techniques that can help you stop smoking during pregnancy. We will explore the benefits of quitting smoking for both you and your baby and provide useful tips to overcome the challenges of nicotine addiction.

Remember, you are not alone in this journey. By making the decision to quit smoking and protect your baby, you are taking a significant step towards ensuring a healthier future for both of you. Let's embark on this transformative journey together and embrace the joy and fulfilment that comes with a smoke-free pregnancy.

Respiratory Issues and Sudden Infant Death Syndrome (SIDS)

In this subchapter, we will delve into the intricacies of respiratory problems that can arise in babies exposed to cigarette smoke in utero. We will explore the links between smoking during pregnancy and the heightened risk of sudden infant death syndrome.

The respiratory system of a developing foetus is vulnerable to the harmful effects of tobacco smoke because it is still in the early stages of growth and development. When a pregnant woman smokes, the chemicals in the smoke, such as nicotine and carbon monoxide, are passed through the placenta and into the baby's bloodstream. These toxic substances can impede the proper development of the baby's lungs and airways.

One of the most common respiratory issues seen in babies exposed to cigarette smoke during pregnancy is a condition known as infant respiratory distress syndrome (IRDS). This condition occurs when the baby's lungs are not fully developed and are unable to produce enough surfactant, a substance that helps keep the air sacs in the lungs open. As a result, the baby may experience difficulty breathing, rapid breathing, and a bluish tint to their skin, known as cyanosis.

Furthermore, exposure to tobacco smoke in utero increases the risk of bronchitis and pneumonia in infants. The chemicals in smoke irritate the delicate lining of the respiratory tract, making it more susceptible to infections. These respiratory infections can be severe and lead to complications such as difficulty breathing and the need for hospitalization.

Another critical concern associated with smoking during pregnancy is the heightened risk of sudden infant death syndrome (SIDS). SIDS is the sudden, unexplained death of a seemingly healthy baby less than one year old. While the exact cause of SIDS remains unknown, research has shown a strong correlation between maternal smoking during pregnancy and an increased risk of SIDS.

Studies have found that babies whose mothers smoke during pregnancy are two to three times more likely to die from SIDS than babies whose mothers do not smoke. The chemicals in tobacco smoke can affect the development of the baby's brainstem, which plays a crucial role in regulating breathing and arousal from sleep. Additionally, smoking during pregnancy may also impair the baby's ability to wake up when faced with decreased oxygen levels, further increasing the risk of SIDS.

It is important to note that the risks associated with smoking during pregnancy are not limited to active smoking alone. Second-hand smoke exposure can also have detrimental effects on the baby's respiratory health and increase the risk of SIDS. When a pregnant woman is exposed to second-hand smoke, the same harmful toxins are present in the air. These toxins can easily pass through the placenta and affect the baby's developing respiratory system.

Given the severe consequences of smoking during pregnancy on the respiratory health of the baby, it is crucial for expectant mothers to quit smoking or avoid exposure to second-hand smoke entirely. Quitting smoking may seem challenging, but it is undoubtedly the best and most effective way to protect your baby's respiratory health and reduce the risk of SIDS.

There are numerous resources available to help pregnant women quit smoking, including support groups, counselling, and nicotine replacement therapy. It is important to reach out to healthcare professionals who specialize in smoking cessation during pregnancy for guidance and support. They can provide personalized advice based on your individual circumstances and help you develop a plan to successfully quit smoking.

In addition to quitting smoking, there are other steps pregnant women can take to further protect their baby's respiratory health. These precautions include creating a smoke-free environment at home by banning smoking indoors and asking family members and visitors to refrain from smoking around you. It is vital to maintain good indoor air quality, ensuring proper ventilation and using air purifiers if necessary.

As an expectant mother, it is essential to prioritize the well-being of your baby by quitting smoking and avoiding exposure to second-hand smoke. Seek professional help and support to quit smoking and create a smoke-free environment to give your baby the best possible start in life. By taking these steps, you are not only protecting your baby's respiratory health but also ensuring a healthier future for both of you.

Cognitive and Behavioral Challenges

Cognitive development refers to the growth and enhancement of mental processes such as thinking, learning, and remembering. It encompasses the ability to problem-solve, make decisions, and understand language. On the other hand, behavioral development entails the acquisition and refinement of social, emotional, and psychological skills, including self-control, empathy, and adaptability.

Several scientific studies have investigated the correlation between smoking during pregnancy and its detrimental effects on a child's cognitive and behavioral development. It is important to note that smoking poses a variety of health risks for both the mother and the foetus, with nicotine being the primary culprit. Nicotine is a highly addictive substance that not only impacts the physiological aspects of smoking but also affects brain development.

One study conducted by researchers at the University of Bristol in the United Kingdom found that children whose mothers smoked during pregnancy were more likely to suffer from attention deficit disorders (ADD) and attention deficit hyperactivity disorder (ADHD). The study followed over 14,000 children and found that those exposed to tobacco smoke in the womb had a significantly higher risk of developing these conditions compared to their non-exposed counterparts. The researchers hypothesized that the interference of nicotine with the developing brain's chemical signalling pathways may be the underlying cause of this association.

Furthermore, smoking during pregnancy has been linked to an increased risk of learning disabilities in children. A study published in the Journal of Paediatrics examined the academic performance of over 5,000 children and found that those whose mothers smoked during pregnancy were more likely to have difficulties with reading, numeracy, and overall school achievement. The researchers speculated that the toxins present in cigarette smoke may disrupt the neural connections necessary for optimal learning and cognitive functioning.

In addition to cognitive challenges, smoking during pregnancy has also been associated with behavioral issues in children. A study conducted by researchers at the University of Turku in Finland found that prenatal exposure to tobacco smoke was linked to an increased likelihood of developing behavioral problems, including aggression, conduct disorder, and difficulties with social interactions. The researchers suggested that nicotine may alter the development of brain regions responsible for emotional regulation and impulse control, leading to these behavioral disturbances.

It is important to recognize that these studies provide evidence of a correlation between smoking during pregnancy and cognitive and behavioral challenges in children. While correlation does not necessarily imply causation, the findings are consistent across multiple research studies, supporting the hypothesis that smoking during pregnancy can have long-lasting effects on a child's cognitive and behavioral development.

The detrimental impact of smoking on the developing foetus extends beyond the direct physiological effects of nicotine. Cigarette smoke contains thousands of harmful chemicals, including carbon monoxide and heavy metals, which can cross the placenta and negatively affect the developing brain. These substances can impair the growth and function of crucial brain structures, leading to lasting cognitive and behavioral challenges.

It is essential for expectant mothers to understand the potential risks associated with smoking during pregnancy and take proactive steps to protect both themselves and their developing baby. Quitting smoking is the most effective strategy to mitigate these risks. By quitting smoking, mothers can significantly reduce the harmful exposure their child receives and improve the overall health and well-being of themselves and their baby.

Quitting smoking during pregnancy can be challenging, but it is not impossible. It requires dedication, support, and a comprehensive plan. As an author and consultant, I am passionate about helping individuals make positive changes in their lives. In the coming sections of this book, we will delve deeper into practical strategies to quit smoking during pregnancy, emphasizing cognitive-behavioral techniques that have proved effective in smoking cessation.

These cognitive-behavioral strategies focus on identifying and modifying the thoughts, feelings, and behaviours that contribute to smoking. By understanding the psychological triggers and developing new coping mechanisms, pregnant women can tackle the addiction and protect their baby from the harmful effects of tobacco smoke.

Furthermore, we will explore the importance of creating a supportive environment, both at home and in the healthcare system, to facilitate smoking cessation during pregnancy. Quitting smoking is a challenging journey, and having a network of understanding and empathetic individuals can make a significant difference in a woman's ability to quit successfully.

Additionally, we will provide guidance on managing stress and cravings, as these are common obstacles that pregnant women face when trying to quit smoking. Understanding how to navigate these challenges effectively can empower women to overcome the addiction and prioritize their baby's health.

The emotional and mental health of a pregnant woman plays a crucial role in ensuring a healthy pregnancy and the overall well-being of both the mother and the baby. Smoking during pregnancy not only poses physical risks but also takes a toll on the emotional and mental health of the expectant mother.

One of the primary concerns associated with smoking during pregnancy is the increased risk of postpartum depression. Research has shown that women who smoke during pregnancy are more likely to experience symptoms of depression after childbirth. The chemicals present in cigarettes, such as nicotine and carbon monoxide, not only affect the physical health of the mother and the baby but also have a profound impact on their mental well-being.

Postpartum depression is a serious condition that can interfere with the mother's ability to bond with her baby, affect her daily functioning, and potentially lead to long-term mental health issues. It is important for expectant mothers to be aware of the potential risks and take proactive steps to quit smoking and protect their emotional well-being.

In addition to postpartum depression, smoking during pregnancy can also increase the risk of anxiety disorders. Anxiety disorders are characterized by excessive worry, fear, and negative emotions that can significantly impact a woman's ability to cope with the challenges of pregnancy and motherhood.

Nicotine, the addictive substance found in cigarettes, acts as a stimulant and can trigger anxiety symptoms in pregnant women. Research has shown that smoking during pregnancy can increase the likelihood of developing anxiety disorders both during and after pregnancy. These disorders can manifest as panic attacks, social anxiety, and generalized anxiety, making it crucial for expectant mothers to quit smoking and seek support to protect their mental well-being.

Furthermore, smoking during pregnancy can also contribute to other psychological challenges, such as low self-esteem and feelings of guilt. Many women who smoke during pregnancy may experience a sense of shame and guilt associated with their habit, which can further exacerbate their emotional and mental distress.

The societal stigma surrounding smoking during pregnancy can create a significant psychological burden for expectant mothers, impacting their self-worth and confidence. It is essential for pregnant women to receive support and understanding from their healthcare providers, family, and friends to address these emotional challenges and develop a positive mindset towards quitting smoking.

Quitting smoking during pregnancy is not easy, and many women may face difficulty in overcoming their addiction. However, seeking help from healthcare professionals, support groups, and counselling services can significantly increase the chances of successfully quitting and protecting both the physical and emotional health of the mother and the baby.

Research has shown that women who receive support and counselling during their quit journey have higher chances of remaining smoke-free throughout pregnancy and beyond. Additionally, behavioral therapies and nicotine replacement therapies can assist in managing withdrawal symptoms and cravings, ensuring a smoother transition to a smoke-free life.

It is crucial for pregnant women to prioritize their emotional well-being during this transformative period of their lives. By focusing on their mental health, expectant mothers can mitigate the potential risks associated with smoking during pregnancy and create the best possible environment for their baby's growth and development.

Chapter 2: Preparing for Quitting

Setting Your Quit Date

Choosing a quit date is undoubtedly a crucial step in the journey to quit smoking. It serves as a concrete starting point from which you can build your path to success. While quitting smoking may seem like an overwhelming task, having a specific date in mind can help you focus your efforts and create a clear roadmap towards achieving your goal.

The first step in setting your quit date is to take a moment to reflect on your personal circumstances and motivations. Ask yourself, why do you want to quit smoking? Is it for your own health? Is it to protect the health of your unborn baby? Understanding the reasons behind your decision will help you stay motivated and committed throughout the quitting process.

Once you have identified your motivations, it's time to choose a quit date that aligns with your goals and priorities. It is important to select a date that allows you ample time to mentally and emotionally prepare for the journey ahead. Quitting smoking is not an easy task, and it requires dedication and perseverance. By giving yourself sufficient time to prepare, you are setting yourself up for success.

Consider selecting a quit date that holds a special significance for you. It could be a meaningful occasion like your birthday or an anniversary, or it could be a meaningful date in relation to your pregnancy journey. Having a date that is personally meaningful can provide you with an extra push of motivation and give you a sense of purpose as you embark on this life-changing journey.

While it is important to choose a quit date that is tailored to your own circumstances, there are a few general guidelines that can help you make an informed decision. It is advisable to avoid selecting a date that coincides with particularly stressful or challenging periods in your life. Instead, aim for a time when you feel relatively calm and stable. By doing so, you can minimize external factors that may contribute to increased cravings or hinder your progress.

It is also essential to ensure that you have a support system in place before your quit date. Quitting smoking is not an easy task, and having a strong support system can make a significant difference in your quitting journey. Reach out to your partner, close friends, or family members and let them know about your decision to quit smoking. Their encouragement, understanding, and accountability can help you stay on track and provide the emotional support you need during challenging moments.

On your quit date, it is important to mentally prepare yourself for the journey ahead. Take some time to reflect on the reasons why you want to quit smoking and remind yourself of all the benefits that await you and your unborn baby. Be proud of the courage and commitment you have shown by making this decision, and use that pride to fuel your determination to succeed.

Removing smoking-related items from your environment can also be a helpful step in mentally preparing for your quit date. Get rid of ashtrays, lighters, and cigarettes, ensuring that you eliminate all physical reminders of your smoking habit. This will not only reduce the temptation to smoke but also serve as a visual representation of your commitment to quit.

As the day progresses, it is essential to keep yourself occupied and distracted from any withdrawal symptoms or cravings that may arise. Engage in activities that you enjoy, such as going for walks, reading a book, practicing deep breathing exercises, or immersing yourself in a hobby that brings you joy. By keeping your mind and body active, you are less likely to dwell on the desire to smoke.

Remember, quitting smoking is a journey, and setbacks may occur along the way. It is crucial to approach these setbacks with resilience and determination rather than viewing them as failures. If you do experience a slip-up, don't be too hard on yourself. Instead, use it as an opportunity to reflect on what triggered the lapse and identify strategies to prevent it from happening again in the future.

In summary, setting a specific quit date is an integral part of the process of quitting smoking during pregnancy. By choosing a date that aligns with your goals, motivations, and personal circumstances, you are setting yourself up for success. Remember to mentally prepare yourself for the journey ahead, remove smoking-related items from your environment, and rely on your support system for encouragement and accountability. With each passing day, you move closer to providing a healthier environment for your unborn baby and embracing a smoke-free life for yourself.

Building a Support Network

Quitting smoking is undoubtedly challenging, especially during pregnancy when the stakes are higher. The cravings, withdrawal symptoms, and the constant battle with addiction can feel overwhelming at times. However, I firmly believe that no one should face this journey alone. Having a support network not only provides a solid foundation for your quit journey but also ensures the emotional and psychological well-being of both you and your baby.

Research has shown that individuals who have a robust support system are more likely to succeed in their goal to quit smoking. In fact, a study published in the British Journal of Health Psychology found that pregnant women who received support from their partners, family, and friends were twice as likely to quit smoking compared to those who did not have any support. This emphasizes the importance of building a support network that nurtures and encourages you throughout this significant phase of your life.

Identifying the right individuals to be a part of your support network is vital. You need individuals who are committed, understanding, and empathetic towards your journey. Here are some key roles you should consider when building your support network:

1. Partner or Spouse:

Your partner or spouse is perhaps the most critical person in your support network. They share your journey, understand your struggles, and are invested in the well-being of both you and your baby. Having open and honest communication with your partner can strengthen your bond and provide a solid foundation of support. They can provide encouragement, hold you accountable, and be a listening ear during challenging moments. By involving your partner, you not only strengthen your relationship but also create a united front against smoking.

2. Family and Friends:

Your family and friends form the backbone of your support system. These are the individuals who know you best and care deeply about your well-being. Sharing your goals and aspirations with them can help create a sense of accountability, providing the motivation needed to stay committed to your journey. Their emotional support and encouragement can make all the difference on days when quitting feels particularly difficult. Make sure to surround yourself with those who are non-judgmental and offer a nurturing environment.

3. Healthcare Professionals:

Your healthcare team, including your obstetrician, midwife, or doula, play a crucial role in your journey to stop smoking during pregnancy. These professionals have the medical knowledge and expertise to guide you through the process and provide essential support and resources. Schedule regular check-ups and consultations to keep them updated on your progress and seek their advice on managing withdrawal symptoms or finding alternative coping mechanisms.

4. Support Groups:

Joining a support group specifically tailored for pregnant women who are quitting smoking can be incredibly beneficial. These groups provide a safe space for you to share your experiences, learn from others who are going through a similar journey, and receive guidance from experts in smoking cessation. Being surrounded by individuals who understand and empathize with your struggles can provide a sense of belonging and help you feel less alone in your journey.

5. Online Communities:

In today's digital age, online communities have become a valuable resource for individuals seeking support and guidance. Joining online forums or social media groups dedicated to pregnant women who are quitting smoking can provide a wealth of information, support, and encouragement. However, always ensure that the information you receive online is from reliable and credible sources.

Building a strong support network is not just about having individuals who cheer you on; it also involves setting boundaries with those who may hinder your progress. It is crucial to distance yourself from people who continue to smoke or enable your smoking habits. Surrounding yourself with positivity and individuals who are committed to your well-being is essential for your success.

Once you have identified the individuals who will be a part of your support network, it is important to communicate your needs and expectations. Let them know what type of support you require, whether it is a daily check-in, words of encouragement, or even distractions when cravings strike. Being open and honest about your vulnerabilities can help foster a supportive environment.

Remember, building a support network is a dynamic process. As your journey progresses, you may find that certain individuals become more valuable in your support system, while others may not provide the support you hoped for. Regularly evaluate your network and make necessary adjustments to ensure you have the optimal support to help you quit smoking and protect the health of your baby.

In conclusion, having a strong support network is essential for pregnant women who are quitting smoking. The journey towards quitting can be challenging, but with the right individuals providing emotional support, accountability, and encouragement, it becomes more manageable. Your partner, family, friends, healthcare professionals, support groups, and online communities can all play vital roles in your support network. Be sure to communicate your needs and expectations to each member, and remember to consistently evaluate and adjust your network as needed. With a strong support network by your side, you can confidently take steps towards a smoke-free future, ensuring the health and well-being of both yourself and your baby.

Creating a Quitting Plan

Quitting smoking can be challenging, especially when you are pregnant and going through hormonal changes. However, with the right strategies and support, you can overcome this addiction and provide your baby with a healthier future. Let's explore some effective techniques that can assist you in your journey to quit smoking.

Step 1: Commitment and Motivation

The first step in creating your quitting plan is to have a strong commitment and motivation to quit smoking.

Reflect on the reasons why you want to quit. Is it because you want to safeguard your baby's health, improve your own health, or set a positive example for your child? Whatever your reasons may be, write them down and keep them in a place where you can see them every day. This will serve as a constant reminder of why you are quitting and help you stay motivated throughout the process.

Step 2: Set a Quit Date

Setting a quit date is an important milestone in your journey towards becoming smoke-free. Choose a date within the next two weeks to give yourself enough time to prepare and get mentally ready. It is essential to pick a day that is relatively stress-free and devoid of any major events or triggers that may tempt you to smoke. On this day, you will make a commitment to yourself and your baby to stop smoking.

Step 3: Gather Support

Having a strong support system is crucial to quit smoking successfully. Reach out to your partner, family, and friends, and share your decision to quit smoking with them. Explain how their support can make a significant difference in your journey. Their encouragement can provide you with the strength and motivation to stay on track. Additionally, consider joining a support group or seeking the guidance of a healthcare professional who specializes in smoking cessation during pregnancy.

Step 4: Identify Triggers

Everyone has different triggers that can cause them to crave a cigarette. It is essential to identify the situations, people, or emotions that make you want to smoke. Common triggers for pregnant women may include stress, boredom, social situations, or even the smell of cigarettes. By being aware of these triggers, you can develop strategies to cope with them effectively.

Step 5: Gradual Reduction

Gradually reducing the number of cigarettes, you smoke as a part of your quitting plan can be an effective approach. It allows your body to adjust slowly to the decreasing nicotine levels, making it easier to overcome withdrawal symptoms. Start by setting a limit on the number of cigarettes you will allow yourself to smoke each day. Then, gradually decrease this number over time until you reach your quit date. While this may not be the most suitable method for everyone, it can be a helpful option for some.

Step 6: Nicotine Replacement Therapy (NRT)

Nicotine replacement therapy (NRT) is a safe and effective method to help pregnant women quit smoking. NRT provides your body with controlled doses of nicotine without the harmful chemicals found in cigarettes. There are various NRT options available, including nicotine patches, gum, inhalers, nasal sprays, and lozenges. Consult with your healthcare provider to determine which method is best for you and how to use it correctly during pregnancy.

Step 7: Alternative Coping Mechanisms

Smoking may have served as a coping mechanism for you in the past, but there are healthier alternatives to deal with stress, cravings, and other emotions. Consider exploring alternative coping mechanisms such as deep breathing exercises, meditation, yoga, or engaging in physical activities like walking or swimming. These activities can help you relax, reduce stress, and distract you from the urge to smoke.

Step 8: Modify Your Environment

As you embark on your journey to quit smoking, it is essential to modify your environment to support your efforts. Remove all cigarettes, lighters, and ashtrays from your home, car, and workplace. Clean and freshen up areas that were associated with smoking. Surround yourself with smoke-free environments, and avoid situations or people that might tempt you to smoke. By changing your surroundings, you can reduce the chances of relapsing and strengthen your commitment to quitting.

Step 9: Coping with Withdrawal Symptoms

Withdrawal symptoms are common when quitting smoking, but they are temporary and manageable. Symptoms may include irritability, restlessness, difficulty concentrating, headaches, and cravings. It is crucial to remind yourself that these symptoms are a sign that your body is healing. Keep yourself busy and find healthy distractions to overcome these temporary challenges. Engage in activities you enjoy, spend time with loved ones, or try new hobbies to keep your mind occupied.

Step 10: Celebrating Milestones

Quitting smoking is a significant achievement, and it is important to celebrate your milestones along the way. Set small goals and reward yourself for reaching them. Treat yourself to something you enjoy, such as a massage, a new outfit, or spending quality time with loved ones. Celebrating your progress will reinforce your motivation and remind you of how far you have come.

Creating a personalized quitting plan is essential to stop smoking successfully during pregnancy. By committing to a plan that suits your needs and circumstances, you increase your chances of protecting your baby's health and ensuring a brighter future for both of you. Remember, you are not alone in this journey. Reach out for support, stay motivated, and believe in your ability to quit smoking and provide the best possible environment for your baby's growth and development.

Identifying Triggers and Coping Strategies

One of the most common triggers for smoking cravings during pregnancy is stress. Pregnancy itself brings forth a range of emotions and challenges, and it is only natural to experience stress during this time. However, it is important to recognize that smoking does not alleviate stress; in fact, it often exacerbates it by negatively impacting our health and the health of our baby. Therefore, finding healthy stress management techniques is vital.

One effective coping strategy is deep breathing exercises. When we feel stressed or overwhelmed, we can take a moment to focus on our breath. Closing our eyes, we slowly inhale through our nose, feeling the air filling our lungs, and then exhale through our mouth, releasing any tension or anxiety. This simple yet powerful technique can help us regain control of our emotions and reduce the urge to smoke.

Another coping strategy is engaging in physical activity. Exercise releases endorphins, which are natural mood boosters. Whether it's going for a walk, taking a prenatal yoga class, or swimming, incorporating regular exercise into our routine can not only reduce stress but also distract us from cravings. Additionally, exercise promotes overall well-being and contributes to a healthier, stronger body for both us and our baby.

It is essential to remember that smoking cravings are temporary; they will pass. During these moments, finding healthy distractions can be incredibly helpful. Engaging in activities that we enjoy can divert our attention away from smoking and provide a sense of fulfilment. For instance, if we enjoy reading, we can immerse ourselves in a captivating book. If we have a creative side, we can explore painting, knitting, or any other form of art that brings us joy. By finding enjoyable distractions, we can gradually rewire our brain to associate pleasure with activities that do not involve smoking.

Additionally, seeking support from loved ones is crucial. Our friends, family, and partners can offer understanding and encouragement during this challenging time. Opening up to them about our cravings and struggles can help alleviate our burden, as they may be able to provide valuable advice and motivation. Sharing our journey with others who genuinely care about our well-being can empower us and strengthen our determination to stop smoking.

Moreover, cultivating a strong support network with fellow pregnant women who are also committed to quitting smoking can provide a formidable sense of camaraderie. Attending support groups or connecting with online communities can enable us to share experiences, triumphs, and setbacks with individuals who are going through similar challenges. Together, we can lift each other up and celebrate our victories, knowing that we are not alone in this battle.

However, it is important to note that each person's journey is unique, and what works for one individual may not work for another. Therefore, it is crucial to be patient with ourselves and experiment with different coping strategies until we find what resonates with us.

Another effective coping strategy is replacing the habit of smoking with healthier alternatives. Many expectant mothers find solace in chewing sugar-free gum or munching on carrot sticks when cravings arise. These alternatives not only provide the oral fixation that smoking often fulfils but also contribute to our overall health by providing essential nutrients and reducing the risk of excessive weight gain during pregnancy.

Furthermore, it is crucial to create a positive and smoke-free environment to reduce the triggers that may lead to cravings. Removing smoking paraphernalia, such as lighters and ashtrays, from our surroundings can help diminish the association between our daily routines and smoking. Additionally, avoiding places or situations that remind us of smoking can further aid in breaking the habit.

Cultivating a Positive Mindset

When I made the decision to quit smoking, I realized that having a positive attitude was crucial. It is easy to get bogged down by negative thoughts and doubts about whether quitting is even possible. But by shifting our mindset, we can empower ourselves to overcome the obstacles and enjoy the benefits of a smoke-free life.

One powerful way to build a positive mindset is through self-affirmation. Self-affirmation is the practice of repeating positive statements about oneself and one's abilities. During the quitting process, the mind can often get overwhelmed with self-doubt and negative thoughts. By consciously replacing these negative thoughts with positive affirmations, we can reprogram our minds to believe in our ability to quit and protect our baby's health.

I found it helpful to create a list of affirmations that resonated with me personally. These affirmations reminded me of my strength, my commitment to my baby's well-being, and the joy and freedom I would experience as a non-smoker. Some examples of affirmations that can be useful for pregnant women quitting smoking include:

- I am strong and capable of overcoming this addiction for my baby's sake.

- I deserve a healthy and smoke-free pregnancy.

- I am in control of my choices and choose a smoke-free life for myself and my baby.

- Every day I am getting closer to a healthier life for me and my baby.

Repeating these affirmations daily, especially in moments of weakness or cravings, helped me stay focused and motivated. It reminded me of the bigger picture and the incredible gift I was giving myself and my baby.

Visualization is another powerful technique that can be used to cultivate a positive mindset. Visualization involves creating vivid mental images of a desired outcome. It's like creating a mental movie of the future you want to manifest. When it comes to quitting smoking, visualizing yourself as a non-smoker can be incredibly motivating.

Close your eyes and imagine a smoke-free future. Picture yourself engaging in activities you love, feeling energized, and enjoying the company of your baby without the interference of cigarettes. Visualize the health benefits you and your baby will experience, such as improved lung function and reduced risk of complications. Imagining these positive scenarios can help anchor your motivation and keep your focus on the joy and benefits of a smoke-free life.

Embracing the joy and benefits of a smoke-free life is essential for maintaining a positive mindset. Quitting smoking is not just about giving something up; it's about gaining so much more. As a pregnant woman, quitting smoking means protecting your baby's health, giving them the best start in life. It means freeing yourself from the grip of addiction and regaining control over your life and choices.

Consider the advantages of a smoke-free life, such as improved energy levels, better sleep, and improved overall health. Think about the financial savings and the ability to spend that money on things that bring you and your baby joy. By focusing on these benefits, you can shift your perspective from feeling deprived to feeling empowered and excited about the transformation taking place in your life.

Throughout my own journey, I found it essential to surround myself with positive influences and a support system. Joining a support group or seeking guidance from a healthcare professional can be incredibly beneficial. Connecting with others who have successfully quit smoking during pregnancy can provide inspiration, accountability, and a sense of community.

Lastly, be kind to yourself throughout this process. Quitting smoking is a significant accomplishment, and there may be moments of slip-ups or setbacks. Remember that each moment is a new opportunity to make a healthy choice. Celebrate your victories, no matter how small they may seem, and learn from any challenges that come your way.

Chapter 3: Overcoming Nicotine Addiction

Understanding Nicotine Addiction

Nicotine addiction is a complex process that involves a chemical substance, nicotine, interacting with receptors in the brain. When a person smokes a cigarette, nicotine is rapidly absorbed into the bloodstream and reaches the brain within seconds. Once in the brain, nicotine binds to receptors, triggering the release of various neurotransmitters, such as dopamine, which are responsible for feelings of pleasure and reward.

Over time, the brain becomes accustomed to the presence of nicotine and starts to rely on it to function normally. This is where the cycle of addiction begins. When nicotine levels in the brain decrease, withdrawal symptoms such as irritability, anxiety, difficulty concentrating, and intense cravings start to emerge. These symptoms can be debilitating, making it extremely challenging to quit smoking.

During pregnancy, the impact of nicotine addiction becomes even more crucial to address. Smoking during pregnancy exposes the developing foetus to harmful toxins and chemicals present in cigarettes. Nicotine has been shown to constrict blood vessels, reducing the oxygen and nutrient supply to the baby. Additionally, it increases the risk of premature birth, low birth weight, stillbirth, and sudden infant death syndrome (SIDS).

Understanding the science behind nicotine addiction is important for pregnant women who want to quit smoking. By understanding the chemical processes that occur in the brain and the reasons behind withdrawal symptoms and cravings, women can have a better grasp on what they are experiencing and be better prepared to tackle them.

Withdrawal symptoms can vary from person to person, but some common symptoms include irritability, anxiety, depression, difficulty concentrating, increased appetite, and sleep disturbances. These symptoms typically peak within the first week after quitting and gradually subside over time. It is important for pregnant women to recognize these symptoms as part of the quitting process and to seek support from healthcare professionals and loved ones to help cope with them.

Cravings are another significant aspect of nicotine addiction. They can be intense and overwhelming, making it challenging for pregnant women to resist the urge to smoke. Cravings often occur when a person is triggered by certain situations or emotions associated with smoking, such as stress, socializing, or after a meal. Understanding these triggers and developing coping strategies to deal with cravings can greatly enhance the chances of successfully quitting smoking during pregnancy.

The cycle of addiction can feel like an endless loop, with withdrawal symptoms leading to cravings, and cravings leading to smoking, which then reinforces the addiction. Breaking this cycle requires determination, support, and effective strategies. Pregnant women should consider seeking guidance from healthcare professionals who specialize in smoking cessation during pregnancy. These professionals can provide personalized advice, support, and resources to help navigate the challenges of quitting smoking.

Additionally, pregnant women can benefit from support groups and counselling services specifically tailored to address smoking cessation during pregnancy. These programs provide a safe and non-judgmental environment for women to share their experiences, learn from others who have successfully quit smoking, and gain valuable insights and strategies to overcome their addiction.

Nicotine Replacement Therapy

Quitting smoking during pregnancy is undoubtedly one of the best decisions a mother can make for both her own health and the health of her unborn baby. However, the addiction to nicotine can make this process incredibly challenging. This is where nicotine replacement therapy (NRT) comes in as a valuable tool to help pregnant women quit smoking.

NRT works by providing pregnant women with a controlled amount of nicotine without the harmful toxins found in cigarettes. It can help reduce cravings, withdrawal symptoms, and the overall urge to smoke, making it easier for expectant mothers to quit smoking and protect themselves and their baby from the harmful effects of cigarettes.

One of the most common forms of NRT is nicotine gum. Nicotine gum works by delivering nicotine to the body through the lining of the mouth when chewed. It allows the pregnant woman to control the amount of nicotine she consumes and helps to alleviate cravings. However, it is important to note that nicotine gum should not be chewed like regular gum; instead, it should be held in the mouth until the nicotine is released and then chewed again. This ensures maximum effectiveness of the nicotine and minimizes the risk of side effects.

Another popular form of NRT is the nicotine patch, which is a small, adhesive patch applied to the skin. The patch slowly releases nicotine into the bloodstream throughout the day, reducing cravings and withdrawal symptoms. Pregnant women using the patch should be cautious and follow their doctor's guidance regarding the appropriate dosage, as wearing the patch for too long may lead to excessive nicotine intake. The patch should be applied to a different area of the skin each day to avoid any irritation.

Nicotine inhalers are another option for pregnant women looking to quit smoking. These inhalers closely mimic the hand-to-mouth action of smoking and allow the user to inhale vaporized nicotine. It provides a quick hit of nicotine, relieving cravings instantly. It is important to note that nicotine inhalers should not be used in the same way as traditional cigarettes. Pregnant women should follow the instructions provided and consult with their healthcare provider for proper usage.

Nicotine nasal sprays are also available as an NRT option. These sprays deliver nicotine to the body through nasal passages instead of inhaling it into the lungs. They provide quick relief from cravings and withdrawal symptoms but may cause nasal irritation. Pregnant women should discuss the use of nasal sprays with their healthcare provider, as the risks and benefits should be carefully evaluated.

While NRT can be a helpful tool in quitting smoking during pregnancy, it is important to remember that it is not without risks. Nicotine, even without the toxins found in cigarettes, can still have adverse effects on the developing foetus. Therefore, it is crucial for pregnant women to consult with their healthcare provider before starting any form of NRT. The healthcare provider will be able to assess the risks and benefits based on the individual's specific circumstances and provide the necessary guidance and support.

It is also essential to use NRT as part of a comprehensive smoking cessation plan that includes behavioral and psychosocial support. NRT is not a standalone solution, and combining it with counselling and support groups can significantly increase the chances of successfully quitting smoking during pregnancy. These additional resources can provide pregnant women with the necessary tools and strategies to cope with cravings and manage the emotional and psychological aspects of quitting smoking.

When using NRT during pregnancy, it is crucial to adhere to safe usage guidelines. Pregnant women should follow the recommended dosage and avoid excessive nicotine intake, as it can have detrimental effects on the foetus. Overdosing on nicotine can cause foetal distress, increased heart rate, and adverse effects on the baby's development. Pregnant women should consult with their healthcare provider to determine the appropriate dosage and ensure safe usage

Behavioral Techniques and Cognitive Restructuring

This subchapter will focus on behavioral techniques and cognitive restructuring strategies that can aid pregnant women in overcoming nicotine addiction. In order to successfully quit smoking during pregnancy, it is important to address both the behavioral and cognitive aspects of addiction. By identifying triggers, creating new habits, and reframing thoughts and beliefs, pregnant women can increase their chances of quitting smoking and protecting their baby's health.

1. Identifying Triggers:

One of the first steps in quitting smoking during pregnancy is to identify the triggers that make you reach for a cigarette. Triggers can be situations, emotions, or routines that prompt cravings for nicotine. It is imperative to be aware of these triggers in order to effectively combat them. To identify your triggers, keep a diary where you record each time you smoke and the circumstances surrounding it. Over time, you will begin to see patterns and common triggers that you can then work on avoiding or finding alternative ways to cope with.

2. Creating New Habits:

Once you have identified your triggers, it is important to replace the habit of smoking with healthier habits. This will not only distract you from smoking but also help to rewire your brain and create new neural pathways. Engaging in activities that promote relaxation such as deep breathing exercises, yoga, or taking a walk can be useful when cravings arise. Changing your routine to incorporate new activities or hobbies that do not involve smoking can also be helpful. For example, instead of reaching for a cigarette after a meal, you can try taking a short walk or savoring a piece of fruit.

3. Reframing Thoughts and Beliefs:

The way we think about smoking and our beliefs surrounding it can greatly influence our ability to quit. It is important to challenge and reframe any negative thoughts or beliefs that may be holding you back from quitting smoking. For example, if you find yourself thinking, "I can't quit, I've tried before and failed," challenge that belief by reminding yourself of your ability to change and of the importance of protecting your baby's health. Replace negative thoughts with positive affirmations such as, "I am a strong and capable woman who can quit smoking for the sake of my baby's well-being."

4. Mindfulness and Meditation:

Practicing mindfulness and meditation can be powerful tools in overcoming nicotine addiction during pregnancy. Mindfulness allows you to be fully present in the moment, observing your thoughts and cravings without judgment. By practicing mindfulness, you can develop a greater awareness of your cravings and become better equipped to manage them. Meditation, on the other hand, can help you cultivate a sense of relaxation and inner calm, reducing stress and anxiety, which are often triggers for smoking. Incorporating these practices into your daily routine can provide you with the mental strength and resilience needed to quit smoking for good.

5. Seeking Support:

Quitting smoking is not an easy task, especially during pregnancy. It is important to seek support from your partner, family, friends, and healthcare professionals. Let them know about your decision to quit smoking and ask for their understanding, encouragement, and assistance during this journey. Consider joining a support group or seeking individual counselling to connect with others who are going through a similar experience. These support systems can provide you with the motivation, accountability, and guidance necessary to successfully quit smoking and protect your baby's health.

6. Rewarding Yourself:

Quitting smoking is a significant accomplishment, and it is important to reward yourself for your progress. Set milestones and goals for yourself, and when you achieve them, celebrate your success. Rewards can be simple and inexpensive, such as treating yourself to a relaxing bath, buying a new book, or indulging in a favourite healthy snack. Recognizing and appreciating your efforts will not only boost your self-confidence but also reinforce the positive changes you are making.

Alternative Therapies and Relaxation Techniques

Acupuncture is one such alternative therapy that has gained significant popularity in recent years. Originating from ancient Chinese medicine, acupuncture involves the insertion of thin needles into specific points on the body. These points, also known as acupoints, are believed to be connected to the body's energy pathways, or meridians. By stimulating these acupoints, acupuncture aims to restore balance and promote the body's natural healing process.

Research has shown that acupuncture can be beneficial in reducing nicotine cravings and withdrawal symptoms. A study conducted by the University of Oslo in Norway found that acupuncture was effective in reducing the number of cigarettes smoked per day by pregnant smokers. The study participants received weekly acupuncture sessions over a period of six weeks, and the results showed a significant decrease in cigarette consumption.

In addition to acupuncture, hypnotherapy is another alternative therapy that can be explored by pregnant women looking to quit smoking. Hypnotherapy involves the use of guided relaxation and focused attention to enter a trance-like state. During this state, the hypnotherapist suggests positive affirmations and encourages the individual to visualize themselves as non-smokers.

Numerous studies have demonstrated the potential benefits of hypnotherapy in smoking cessation. A research study conducted by the University of Texas found that pregnant smokers who received hypnotherapy had a higher rate of quitting compared to those who received usual care. The study participants underwent five hypnotherapy sessions tailored specifically for smoking cessation. The findings indicated that hypnotherapy can significantly increase the chances of successful quitting during pregnancy.

Another relaxation technique that can complement the quitting process is deep breathing exercises. Deep breathing involves taking slow, deep breaths in through the nose, allowing the diaphragm to expand, and exhaling slowly through the mouth. This technique promotes relaxation by activating the body's parasympathetic nervous system, which counteracts the effects of stress.

Research studies have shown that deep breathing exercises can effectively reduce anxiety and cravings associated with smoking. A study conducted by the University of California, San Francisco found that pregnant women who practiced deep breathing exercises experienced decreased cravings and improved mood. The deep breathing exercises were incorporated into the participants' daily routines, and they reported a decrease in the urge to smoke throughout the day.

Mindfulness practices are also gaining recognition for their effectiveness in smoking cessation. Mindfulness involves being fully present in the moment, observing thoughts and emotions without judgment. This practice can help individuals become more aware of their smoking habits and the triggers that lead to smoking.

Studies have shown that incorporating mindfulness into smoking cessation programs can lead to increased quitting rates. A research study conducted by the University of Wisconsin-Madison found that pregnant smokers who participated in a mindfulness-based program had higher rates of abstinence compared to those who received a standard care program. The mindfulness program consisted of weekly group sessions where participants learned mindfulness techniques and strategies to cope with cravings.

Incorporating alternative therapies and relaxation techniques into the journey of quitting smoking during pregnancy can be highly beneficial. However, it is essential to consult with healthcare providers before embarking on any alternative therapy to ensure its safety and compatibility with the individual's health condition.

Celebrating Milestones and Staying Motivated

Quitting smoking during pregnancy is a significant milestone in itself, and it should be celebrated and acknowledged. It takes tremendous courage and determination to make such a positive change for both yourself and your baby. Celebrating these milestones not only helps to boost your morale but also serves as a reminder of the progress you have made so far.

One way to celebrate milestones is by rewarding oneself. Each time you reach a significant milestone, whether it's a week, a month, or even a day without smoking, take a moment to acknowledge your achievement. Treat yourself to something special, like a relaxing massage, a favourite meal, or a new outfit. By rewarding yourself, you reinforce the positive decision you have made to quit smoking and create a sense of accomplishment that can motivate you to keep going.

Seeking support from loved ones is another crucial aspect of staying motivated during this journey. Surrounding yourself with people who believe in you and your ability to quit smoking will provide the encouragement and support you need. Share your milestones with your partner, family, and close friends, and let them celebrate with you. Their words of encouragement and acknowledgment can go a long way in boosting your confidence and motivation.

Additionally, consider joining support groups or seeking professional help. These resources can provide a safe space to share your experiences, challenges, and triumphs with others who are going through a similar journey. Connecting with other pregnant women who have successfully quit smoking can be an excellent source of inspiration. Hearing their success stories can reaffirm your belief in your own ability to quit smoking and provide you with practical tips and strategies that have worked for them.

Finding inspiration in success stories is another powerful way to stay motivated throughout your quit smoking journey. Take the time to read stories, watch videos, or listen to podcasts of individuals who have successfully quit smoking during pregnancy. Their stories serve as a reminder that it is indeed possible to overcome this addiction and protect your baby's health. Pay attention to the challenges they faced and the strategies they used to overcome them. Learning from their experiences can provide you with valuable insights that can support your own quit smoking journey.

One success story that particularly resonated with me was that of Emma, a pregnant woman who successfully quit smoking for the well-being of her unborn child. Emma was initially sceptical about her ability to quit smoking, having tried and failed several times in the past. However, when she learned that she was pregnant, she knew that it was the perfect time to make a change for the better.

Emma started her journey by setting small, achievable goals for herself. Instead of trying to quit smoking cold turkey, she gradually reduced the number of cigarettes she smoked each day. She celebrated each milestone, no matter how small, and rewarded herself with something she truly enjoyed. By taking this approach, Emma found that she was able to build up her motivation and gradually increase her confidence in her ability to quit smoking completely.

As Emma progressed in her quit smoking journey, she discovered the importance of seeking support from loved ones. She confided in her partner, who provided unwavering support and encouragement throughout her journey. Emma also reached out to a local support group for pregnant women who were trying to quit smoking, where she found a sense of camaraderie and understanding. The shared experiences and advice from other women in the group served as a constant source of motivation for Emma.

What inspired Emma the most were the success stories she came across during her research. She read about mothers who had successfully quit smoking and witnessed the incredible improvements in their babies' health. These stories served as a reminder of the positive impact quitting smoking can have on both the mother and the baby. Emma was particularly moved by the stories of mothers who had struggled with their addiction but managed to overcome it through sheer determination and the support of their loved ones.

Emma's success story is just one example of the many inspiring stories out there. Each journey is unique, and while there may be challenges along the way, celebrating milestones and staying motivated can make a significant difference. By rewarding yourself, seeking support from loved ones, and finding inspiration in success stories, you are laying the foundation for a smoke-free future for both yourself and your baby.

Remember, quitting smoking is not only a gift to yourself but also a tremendous gift to your baby. By staying motivated and celebrating milestones, you are taking an essential step towards ensuring a healthier and happier future for both of you.

Chapter 4: Creating a Healthy Environment

Removing Smoking Remnants

Smoke residue, also known as thirdhand smoke, is a toxic residue that remains on surfaces even after the visible smoke has dissipated. This residue can be found on walls, furniture, carpets, and even in dust particles. It contains harmful chemicals that can be particularly dangerous for pregnant women and unborn babies.

Cleaning Techniques:

To ensure a smoke-free living environment, it is essential to adopt effective cleaning techniques. Regularly clean your home, paying special attention to areas that may have come into direct contact with smoke. Start by dusting all surfaces, using a damp cloth to prevent the spread of dust particles into the air. Vacuum all carpets and upholstery thoroughly, as these materials tend to retain smoke residue.

When cleaning any hard surfaces such as walls, floors, or countertops, use a mixture of warm water and mild detergent to remove the smoke residue effectively. It is important to avoid using harsh chemicals, as they can potentially worsen the air quality in your home. Opting for natural cleaning solutions or products specifically designed to remove smoke residue can be a safer alternative.

Air Purifiers:

In addition to thorough cleaning, investing in an air purifier can significantly improve the air quality in your home. Air purifiers work by filtering out harmful particles from the air, including smoke residue, dust, and allergens. They can be particularly beneficial in removing the lingering smoke odours and reducing the risk of second-hand smoke exposure.

When selecting an air purifier, ensure that it is equipped with a High-Efficiency Particulate Air (HEPA) filter. HEPA filters are highly effective at capturing even the smallest particles, including smoke residue. Additionally, look for air purifiers that have activated carbon filters, as they can help absorb and neutralize odours.

Place the air purifier in the room where you spend the most time, such as the bedroom or living room. This will help create a safe and clean environment for you and your baby. Remember to regularly clean and change the filters as recommended by the manufacturer to ensure the optimal performance of the air purifier.

Fresh Air Circulation:

While cleaning techniques and air purifiers play a crucial role in removing smoking remnants, fresh air circulation is equally important. Opening windows and allowing fresh air to flow into your living space can help dilute any remaining smoke residue and improve indoor air quality.

Make it a habit to open windows for a few minutes each day, particularly in rooms where you often smoke or where the smoke residue is most prevalent. Additionally, consider using fans or ventilation systems to facilitate air circulation and aid in the removal of smoke particles.

Creating a designated smoking area outside your home can also prevent smoke from entering your living space. This will help contain the smoke residue and reduce the risk of exposure to both you and your baby. Ensure that this smoking area is located far away from any open windows or ventilation systems.

Creating a Supportive Social Circle

Quitting smoking during pregnancy is undoubtedly challenging. It requires a great deal of determination, support, and understanding from those around you.

That's why building a supportive social circle is vital to your success in this journey.

First and foremost, let's address the significance of effective communication with your loved ones. It's important to remember that your friends and family may not fully understand the struggles you face as you quit smoking. They may unintentionally say or do things that could cause distress or trigger cravings. However, it is essential to approach these situations with patience and kindness.

One effective way to communicate with your loved ones is through honest and open conversations. Sit down with them and explain your decision to quit smoking during pregnancy and why it is so important for the health of you and your baby. Share your fears, concerns, and the goals you have set for yourself in your journey towards quitting.

During these conversations, encourage your loved ones to ask questions and express their thoughts and concerns. Be prepared for their reactions, which may range from surprise to scepticism. Remember, they may not fully comprehend the complexities of addiction and the incredible willpower it takes to quit. By educating them and being open to their questions, you can help them understand your perspective and garner their support.

Another essential aspect of building a supportive social circle is seeking understanding. While it is understandable that not everyone will fully grasp the challenges of giving up smoking, empathy and compassion can play a crucial role in creating a supportive environment.

It's important to acknowledge that certain situations and comments might inadvertently trigger cravings and make it harder for you to stay smoke-free. Communicate your needs to your friends and family and seek understanding from them. Let them know if certain conversations or activities are difficult for you and ask if they can avoid discussing or engaging in them around you. By doing so, you can minimize the chances of succumbing to cravings.

Additionally, it is helpful to explore alternative ways of spending time with your loved ones that do not involve smoking or being in situations where smoking is prevalent. Suggest activities such as going for walks, watching movies, or engaging in hobbies that promote a smoke-free environment. By actively seeking out smoke-free activities, you can create a supportive social circle that aligns with your goal of quitting smoking during pregnancy.

Now, let's dive into some strategies that can aid you in avoiding triggering situations. One effective approach is identifying your triggers and developing strategies to avoid or manage them. Triggers can be environmental, social, or emotional cues that increase your desire to smoke. Examples include being around other smokers, feeling stressed or anxious, or being in certain places or situations you associate with smoking.

By identifying your triggers, you can create a plan to proactively avoid them. For instance, if you have friends who smoke, consider reducing your exposure to these situations until you feel more confident in your ability to resist the urge to smoke. If stress is a trigger for you, explore stress management techniques such as deep breathing exercises or engaging in relaxation activities like yoga or meditation.

Preparing a list of alternative activities or distractions can also be beneficial. When a craving hits, having a predetermined plan can help divert your attention away from smoking. Consider engaging in activities that bring you joy and relaxation, such as reading a book, taking a warm bath, or listening to calming music. These distractions can provide a much-needed escape from the craving and help you remain smoke-free.

In addition to avoiding triggering situations, it is equally important to establish a support system that can assist you when cravings arise. This support system can consist of family members, friends, or even support groups where you can share your journey, seek guidance, and celebrate your successes. Surrounding yourself with people who understand and support your decision to quit smoking during pregnancy can be incredibly empowering.

Remember, quitting smoking is a journey, and setbacks are a natural part of that process. Being part of a supportive social circle during these challenging moments can make a world of difference. These individuals can provide you with the encouragement, motivation, and accountability you need to stay the course.

Designing a Relaxing and Stress-Free Space

Aromatherapy: A Journey to Serenity

The sense of smell is incredibly powerful and can evoke vivid memories and emotions. Aromatherapy is a technique that harnesses the power of scents to promote relaxation and reduce stress. By using essential oils and natural fragrances, you can create a soothing ambiance within your home.

One of the most effective ways to incorporate aromatherapy into your space is through the use of diffusers. These devices disperse essential oils into the air, filling the room with calming scents. Lavender, chamomile, and ylang-ylang are popular choices for relaxation and stress relief. These fragrances have been shown to reduce anxiety, promote sleep, and create a sense of tranquillity.

In addition to diffusers, you can also use scented candles or potpourri to infuse your space with soothing aromas. When using candles, make sure to choose natural, non-toxic options, as synthetic fragrances can release harmful chemicals into the air.

opt for soy or beeswax candles with essential oil scents for a healthier alternative.

Soothing Colours: Painting Your World in Calm

Colour has a profound impact on our emotions and can influence our mood and overall well-being. When designing a relaxing and stress-free space, it is important to choose colours that foster a sense of calmness and serenity.

Soft and muted hues are generally more soothing and can create a calming atmosphere. Shades of blue, green, and purple are particularly known for their relaxing properties. These colours are reminiscent of nature and can evoke a sense of tranquillity and peace. Consider painting your walls in these soothing shades or incorporating them through furniture, curtains, and accessories.

Another technique to create a relaxing environment is through the use of colour psychology. This is a discipline that explores the psychological effects of colour on human behaviour. For example, blue is known to promote relaxation and reduce stress, while yellow can enhance optimism and joy. By understanding the psychological impact of different colours, you can strategically incorporate them into your space to achieve the desired effect.

Comfortable Furniture Arrangements: Nurturing Your Body and Soul

Creating a stress-free space goes beyond just aesthetics. It also involves designing a functional and comfortable environment that nurtures both your body and soul. One of the key aspects of this is choosing the right furniture and arranging it in a way that promotes relaxation and ease.

When selecting furniture, opt for pieces that prioritize comfort and support. During pregnancy, your body undergoes numerous changes, and it is important to have furniture that accommodates these transformations. Consider investing in a comfortable and supportive chair or sofa where you can relax and unwind.

In addition to choosing the right furniture, consider the arrangement of the pieces within the space. A cluttered and disorganized environment can add to feelings of stress and unease. On the other hand, a well-planned and organized space promotes a sense of calmness and serenity.

Arrange your furniture in a way that allows for easy movement and flow within the room. Avoid placing furniture in high-traffic areas where it may obstruct movement. Create cozy nooks and designated relaxation areas where you can retreat and unwind.

Incorporating Other Elements of Relaxation

Creating a relaxing and stress-free space is not limited to aromatherapy, soothing colours, and comfortable furniture arrangements. There are numerous other elements you can incorporate to enhance the overall ambiance and promote relaxation.

Soft lighting is an essential component of a calming environment. Harsh or bright lights can be jarring and increase feelings of tension. opt for warm, dimmable lighting options that create a soft and cozy atmosphere. Use lamps and dimmer switches to have more control over the lighting in your space.

Natural elements such as plants can also contribute to a tranquil environment. Not only do they add a touch of beauty to your space, but they also purify the air and create a connection with nature. Choose plants that are low-maintenance and safe for your space. Snake plants, peace lilies, and pothos are great options for beginners.

Finally, incorporating relaxation techniques such as meditation and mindfulness can further enhance the tranquillity of your space. Set aside a designated area for meditation or mindfulness practice, where you can escape the outside world and focus on your well-being. Use cushions or comfortable seating arrangements to create a space that promotes relaxation and introspection.

Designing a relaxing and stress-free space is a vital step in your journey to stop smoking during pregnancy and protect your baby. By incorporating techniques such as aromatherapy, soothing colours, and comfortable furniture arrangements, you can create an environment that supports your physical and emotional well-being. Remember, your space should be a sanctuary—a place where you can escape the stresses of the outside world and focus on nurturing yourself and your baby.

Incorporating Healthy Habits

Here, we will discuss the importance of incorporating healthy habits into daily life to support the quitting process. We will explore topics such as regular exercise, nutritious diet choices, and engaging in activities that promote relaxation and self-care.

I believe that incorporating healthy habits into our daily lives is essential not only for quitting smoking but also for overall well-being. When you are pregnant, it becomes even more crucial to prioritize your health and take care of your body. Quitting smoking is a significant step in the right direction, and by incorporating healthy habits, you can further enhance the benefits for both yourself and your baby.

1. Regular Exercise:

Regular exercise has been proven to have numerous health benefits, including alleviating stress and boosting mood. When it comes to quitting smoking during pregnancy, exercise can play a pivotal role in managing cravings and preventing weight gain. Engaging in physical activity not only distracts you from the urge to smoke but also releases endorphins, which help in elevating your mood.

It is essential to choose exercises that are safe and suitable for pregnancy. Consult with your healthcare provider before starting any exercise regimen to ensure that it aligns with your specific needs and limitations. Low-impact exercises such as walking, swimming, and prenatal yoga are generally safe options for pregnant women.

Remember, even light exercise can make a significant difference. Start slowly and gradually increase the intensity or duration of your workouts to avoid overexertion. Aim for at least 30 minutes of moderate exercise most days of the week, but listen to your body and adjust accordingly. Be gentle with yourself and enjoy the process of moving your body in a way that feels good and supports your overall well-being.

2. Nutritious Diet Choices:

A nutritious diet is crucial for the health of both you and your baby during pregnancy. By consuming a well-balanced diet, you are providing essential nutrients for the growth and development of your child, while also supporting your own health. When quitting smoking, a nutritious diet can be particularly beneficial in managing cravings and minimizing weight gain.

During pregnancy, it is important to focus on consuming nutrient-rich foods that provide adequate protein, calcium, iron, folic acid, and other essential vitamins and minerals. Incorporate a variety of fruits, vegetables, whole grains, lean proteins, and low-fat dairy products into your daily meals. Avoid processed foods, sugary snacks, and excessive caffeine, as they can negatively impact your health and make it more challenging to quit smoking.

Remember that making dietary changes should be a gradual process. Start by identifying any unhealthy eating habits and replacing them with healthier alternatives. Find creative ways to make nutritious meals enjoyable and satisfying. Seek guidance from a registered dietitian who can help you create a

customized meal plan that meets your nutritional
needs during pregnancy.

3. Engaging in Activities that Promote Relaxation
and Self-Care:

Quitting smoking can be a stressful and challenging
journey, especially during pregnancy when hormones
and emotions are already heightened. Engaging in
activities that promote relaxation and self-care can
significantly support your efforts to quit smoking and
maintain a positive mindset throughout the process.

Find activities that help you relax and unwind, such
as meditation, deep breathing exercises, or taking a
warm bath. These techniques can help reduce stress,
improve sleep quality, and provide a sense of calm
when cravings arise.

Additionally, prioritize self-care activities that make
you feel good and nurture your overall well-being.
This can include activities such as reading a book,
listening to soothing music, practicing mindfulness,
or getting a prenatal massage. Take the time to
pamper yourself and indulge in activities that help
you reconnect with yourself and your body.

It is also essential to surround yourself with a support
system that understands your journey and encourages
your efforts to quit smoking. Seek the support of
loved ones, friends, and professionals who can offer
guidance, motivation, and accountability along the
way.

Incorporating healthy habits into your daily life is not
only beneficial during pregnancy but sets the
foundation for a healthier future for both you and
your baby. By prioritizing regular exercise, nutritious
diet choices, and activities that promote relaxation
and self-care, you are not only supporting your
quitting journey but also cultivating a lifestyle that
promotes overall wellness.

Remember, quitting smoking during pregnancy is the best gift you can give to yourself and your baby. By incorporating healthy habits into your daily routine, you are taking proactive steps to ensure a healthier and brighter future for both of you. Embrace the process, be kind to yourself, and celebrate each small victory along the way. You are stronger than you think, and with the right support and healthy habits, you can successfully quit smoking and protect your baby's health.

Seeking Professional Help and Resources

As an expectant mother, the decision to quit smoking is not an easy one. The addiction to nicotine can be powerful, and the withdrawal symptoms can make it even more challenging. However, seeking professional help can greatly increase your chances of success. Healthcare providers, such as doctors, midwives, and obstetricians, play a crucial role in providing assistance and guidance throughout the journey of quitting smoking during pregnancy.

One of the first steps in seeking professional help is to schedule an appointment with your healthcare provider to discuss your smoking habits and your desire to quit. They can provide you with valuable insights into the effects of smoking during pregnancy and the benefits of quitting for both you and your baby. Additionally, they can offer various treatment options and support services tailored to your specific needs.

Healthcare providers can prescribe nicotine replacement therapy (NRT) or other medications to help ease the cravings and withdrawal symptoms associated with quitting smoking. NRT comes in various forms, such as patches, gum, lozenges, inhalers, and nasal sprays. These products deliver controlled amounts of nicotine to the body, reducing the urge to smoke while avoiding the harmful chemicals found in cigarettes.

Furthermore, doctors can refer you to specialized cessation programs or clinics that focus on helping pregnant women quit smoking. These programs often offer a combination of counselling, behavioral therapy, and medication, increasing the chances of long-term success in smoking cessation. Through these programs, you will not only receive professional support but also have access to a network of individuals going through a similar journey, providing a sense of community and understanding.

Another valuable resource in quitting smoking during pregnancy is support groups. Support groups bring together individuals who are facing similar challenges and provide a platform for sharing experiences, offering advice, and providing emotional support. Many healthcare facilities offer support group sessions specifically for pregnant women who want to quit smoking. These sessions are often led by healthcare professionals with expertise in smoking cessation.

In a support group, you will have the opportunity to hear other women's stories, learn from their journey, and gain valuable insights into the obstacles they faced and how they overcame them. Moreover, being part of a support group creates a sense of accountability as you share your progress and set goals in a non-judgmental and supportive environment.

In addition to physical support groups, online forums and communities can also provide immense support and guidance during the quitting process. Online platforms offer the convenience of connecting with others from the comfort of your own home, allowing you to access information, seek advice, and share experiences at any time of the day.

There are several reputable online forums and websites dedicated to helping pregnant women quit smoking. These platforms often include discussion boards, chat rooms, and resources that provide evidence-based information on quitting smoking during pregnancy. The opportunity to connect with a broader community of women who share similar goals and struggles can be immensely beneficial in staying motivated and overcoming challenges along the way.

Moreover, online resources can provide access to educational materials, interactive tools, and even virtual counselling sessions with healthcare professionals specializing in smoking cessation for pregnant women. These resources are designed to empower and equip expectant mothers with the knowledge and tools needed to successfully quit smoking and maintain a smoke-free life during pregnancy.

Chapter 5: Managing Cravings and Withdrawal Symptoms

Identifying Triggers and Distracting Techniques

Here, we will discuss effective methods to identify triggers that may lead to smoking cravings and provide distraction techniques to divert attention away from the urge to smoke. We will explore options such as engaging in hobbies, practicing mindfulness, and seeking support from loved ones. By understanding your triggers and adopting healthy distraction methods, you can successfully quit smoking and protect your baby's well-being.

1. Understanding Triggers

Smoking cravings often arise due to certain triggers in our environment, emotions, or behaviours. It is crucial to identify these triggers to better control and overcome the urge to smoke. Triggers can vary from person to person, but common ones include stress, social situations, certain places, and specific activities. By pinpointing these triggers, you can develop strategies to avoid or manage them effectively.

One helpful exercise is to keep a journal to track your smoking cravings and identify patterns. Take note of the time, location, and emotional state when the cravings arise. Over time, you may notice recurring triggers, such as feeling stressed during work hours or experiencing cravings in social gatherings. This awareness will enable you to be more proactive in avoiding or finding alternative coping mechanisms for these triggers.

2. Engaging in Hobbies and Activities

Engaging in hobbies or activities that you enjoy can be an excellent distraction from smoking cravings.

Immersing yourself in an enjoyable task not only provides a temporary escape from the urge to smoke but also helps to rewire your brain and establish new, healthy habits. Consider the following hobbies and activities that can be particularly effective:

a) Exercise: Physical exercise releases endorphins, which elevate mood and reduce cravings. It also increases oxygen flow and improves overall well-being. Choose activities that suit your fitness level and preferences, such as walking, swimming, or prenatal yoga. Not only will exercise distract you from the urge to smoke, but it will also benefit your overall health, as well as your baby's development.

b) Creative pursuits: Engaging in creative outlets, such as painting, writing, or playing a musical instrument, can be highly therapeutic and distracting. These activities channel your focus and energy into something productive, diverting your attention away from smoking cravings. Moreover, the sense of accomplishment and joy it brings can boost your confidence and motivate you to continue staying smoke-free.

c) Cooking and baking: Experimenting with new recipes and spending time in the kitchen can be an enjoyable and effective way to distract yourself from smoking cravings. Preparing nutritious meals not only provides a healthier alternative to smoking but also nurtures your body and nourishes your baby. Take advantage of this time to explore healthy and delicious recipes that will further support your commitment to a smoke-free lifestyle.

3. Practicing Mindfulness and Stress Reduction Techniques

Mindfulness techniques can be powerful tools to manage cravings and reduce stress. Mindfulness involves being fully present in the moment, without judgment or attachment to thoughts or emotions. By cultivating mindfulness, you can observe your cravings objectively and let them pass without feeling overwhelmed or compelled to smoke. Consider the following mindfulness exercises:

a) Deep breathing: Deep, slow breathing triggers the relaxation response and promotes a sense of calm. Practice deep breathing exercises whenever you feel a craving arising, focusing on your breath as it goes in and out. This simple technique helps redirect your attention away from smoking and brings you back to the present moment.

b) Meditation: Regular meditation practice can significantly reduce stress and increase self-awareness, making it an effective tool for managing smoking cravings. Find a comfortable and quiet space, close your eyes, and focus on your breath or a specific mantra or visualization. Allow your thoughts to come and go without judgment, gently bringing your attention back to your chosen point of focus. Through consistent practice, you will develop a greater ability to detach from cravings and regain control over your actions.

c) Progressive muscle relaxation: Progressive muscle relaxation involves systematically tensing and then relaxing each muscle group in your body. This technique promotes physical and mental relaxation, helping to reduce stress and cravings. Start by tensing and releasing your toes, and gradually work your way up through your legs, abdomen, chest, arms, and face. As you actively engage your muscles and then release the tension, you will experience a deep sense of relaxation and calmness.

4. Seeking Support from Loved Ones

Quitting smoking during pregnancy can be challenging, but having a strong support system can make all the difference. Reach out to your loved ones, friends, and family members who are aware of your decision to quit smoking. Share your struggles and cravings with them, as they can provide encouragement, understanding, and practical advice.

Consider joining support groups specifically designed for pregnant women who are quitting smoking. These groups provide a safe space to share experiences, gain insights, and receive support from individuals who are going through similar challenges. Additionally, counselling or therapy sessions with professionals experienced in smoking cessation during pregnancy can further enhance your chances of success.

Remember that quitting smoking is not a journey you have to face alone. Reach out and lean on your support network whenever you need guidance or a listening ear. Their unwavering support and encouragement will empower you to stay committed to your goal of protecting your baby's health.

Healthy Alternatives to Smoking

Chewing Sugar-Free Gum:

One of the easiest and most accessible alternatives to smoking is chewing sugar-free gum. When you feel the urge to smoke, popping in a piece of gum can help distract your mind and provide oral stimulation. The act of chewing gum can also help reduce anxiety and stress, which are commonly associated with cravings. Additionally, many sugar-free gums contain ingredients like xylitol, which can help prevent tooth decay—a common issue during pregnancy. However, it is important to note that excessive consumption of sugar-free gum may have a laxative effect, so it is best to chew it in moderation.

Snacking on Fruits and Vegetables:

Another healthy alternative to smoking is snacking on fruits and vegetables. Not only do they provide a burst of flavour, but they are also packed with essential vitamins and minerals that are vital for the health of both the mother and the baby. Fruits and vegetables can help satisfy cravings while also providing fibre, which can promote healthy digestion—a common issue during pregnancy.

Additionally, snacking on these nutritious foods can help prevent unnecessary weight gain, which is another concern during pregnancy. Some fruits and vegetables that are particularly beneficial for pregnant women include bananas, carrots, apples, oranges, and cucumbers. These snacks are not only convenient to carry around, but they also provide a refreshing and healthy alternative to smoking.

Engaging in Physical Activities:

Engaging in physical activities can be an excellent way to distract your mind from smoking cravings while also benefiting your overall health during pregnancy. Regular exercise is not only safe for most pregnant women but is also highly recommended by healthcare professionals. Exercise releases endorphins, which are natural mood boosters, helping to reduce stress and anxiety—two common triggers for smoking cravings. Additionally, staying active during pregnancy can help improve blood circulation, increase energy levels, and promote better quality sleep. However, it is important to consult with your healthcare provider before starting any exercise routine to ensure it is safe for you and your baby.

There are various types of physical activities you can engage in during pregnancy, depending on your fitness level and personal preferences. Walking is a popular and low-impact exercise that can be easily incorporated into your daily routine. Consider taking regular walks in your neighbourhood or exploring nearby parks for a change of scenery. Swimming and prenatal yoga are also great options for pregnant women, as they both provide gentle workouts with minimal impact on the joints. These activities can not only help you manage cravings but can also provide an opportunity for relaxation and self-care.

In addition to these healthier alternatives, it is important to develop coping mechanisms that can be used in moments of intense cravings. Here are a few strategies that can help:

1. Deep Breathing: Taking slow, deep breaths can help calm your mind and reduce cravings. Inhale deeply through your nose, hold your breath for a few seconds, and exhale slowly through your mouth. Repeat this several times until you feel more relaxed.

2. Distraction Techniques: Finding activities that can keep your mind occupied can be effective in managing cravings. Engaging in hobbies, reading a book, or watching a movie can help divert your attention away from smoking.

3. Support Network: Surrounding yourself with a supportive network of friends, family, or a support group can make a significant difference in your journey to quit smoking. Sharing your struggles, celebrating your successes, and seeking encouragement from others who have been through similar experiences can provide invaluable support.

4. Journaling: Keeping a journal can act as a therapeutic tool to vent your emotions and track your progress. It can also serve as a reminder of the reasons why you want to quit smoking and the positive changes you are making for yourself and your baby.

Relaxation Techniques and Stress Management

One of the key techniques we will focus on is deep breathing exercises. Deep breathing is a simple yet powerful tool that can help you relax and regain control of your emotions. When we are stressed or experiencing cravings, our breathing tends to become shallow and rapid. By consciously practicing deep breathing, we can slow down our breath and activate the body's relaxation response.

To get started, find a quiet and comfortable place where you can sit or lie down. Close your eyes and take a moment to become aware of your breath. Begin by taking a slow and deep breath in through your nose, filling your lungs with air. Feel your abdomen expand as you inhale. Hold your breath for a few seconds, and then exhale slowly through your mouth, releasing all the air from your lungs. Repeat this process several times, allowing each breath to become slower and deeper. As you focus on your breath, imagine the smoke leaving your body and being replaced with fresh, clean air. Feel the tension in your body dissipate with each exhale. Practice this deep breathing exercise whenever you feel stressed or overwhelmed, and incorporate it into your daily routine to cultivate a sense of calm and relaxation.

Another effective technique for managing stress and cravings is progressive muscle relaxation (PMR). PMR involves systematically tensing and releasing different muscle groups in your body to promote physical and mental relaxation. This technique helps you become more aware of the tension in your muscles and teaches you how to release it, promoting a sense of peace and tranquillity.

To practice PMR, find a quiet and comfortable space where you can lie down. Start by tensing the muscles in your toes and feet as tightly as you can, holding the tension for a few seconds, and then releasing it completely. Move up to your calves and thighs, contracting and relaxing each muscle group. Continue this process, working your way up through your abdomen, chest, arms, and finally, your face and scalp. As you release the tension in each muscle group, focus on the sensation of relaxation and imagine the stress and cravings flowing out of your body. Practice PMR daily, especially during times of heightened stress or when cravings are particularly strong, to help you stay cantered and focused on your smoke-free journey.

In addition to deep breathing exercises and progressive muscle relaxation, journaling can be a powerful tool for managing stress and cravings. Writing down your thoughts and feelings allows you to gain clarity and perspective, helping you identify triggers and develop effective coping strategies. Journaling also provides a safe and private outlet for expressing your emotions, reducing the risk of bottling up your feelings, which can increase stress levels.

To begin your journaling practice, set aside a few minutes each day to reflect on your experiences and feelings. Start by jotting down any cravings or stressors you may have faced throughout the day. Explore the emotions associated with these triggers and write about how you managed them. Did you engage in any specific techniques, such as deep breathing or PMR? Did you reach out to a support system? By documenting your thoughts and actions, you can track your progress and identify patterns in your cravings and reactions to stress. Additionally, you can use journaling as a platform for setting goals, expressing gratitude, and celebrating your victories, no matter how small. Remember, every step forward is a step towards a healthier you and a healthier baby.

Aside from the specific techniques mentioned above, it is important to incorporate self-care activities into your daily routine. Pregnancy can be a wonderful yet challenging time, and taking care of your physical, emotional, and mental well-being is crucial. Engage in activities that bring you joy and relaxation. This could include taking gentle walks, practicing prenatal yoga, listening to calming music, or indulging in a warm bubble bath. Prioritize quality sleep and ensure you are eating a balanced diet to support your overall health and well-being.

Supportive Communication and Accountability

One of the most powerful tools we have in overcoming any challenge is effective communication. When it comes to quitting smoking during pregnancy, supportive communication is even more crucial to ensure a successful journey. As expectant mothers, we may face a unique set of physical and emotional challenges, and having the support of our loved ones can make all the difference.

When I decided to quit smoking during my wife's pregnancy, I knew that it was not going to be an easy journey. However, I was fortunate enough to have the love and support of my wife, family, and friends, which made the process more manageable. Their understanding and encouragement helped me stay accountable to my decision, and their words of encouragement acted as a constant reminder of why I was making this sacrifice.

If you are in a similar situation, it is essential to communicate your decision to your loved ones and help them understand why quitting smoking is so important for both you and your unborn baby. Explain to them the risks and dangers associated with smoking during pregnancy, and share your personal reasons for wanting to quit. By doing so, you will create an environment of understanding and empathy, enabling your loved ones to provide the support you need.

It can be helpful to have an open and honest conversation with your partner, as they will likely be your primary source of support throughout this journey. Share your concerns, fears, and challenges with them, and ask for their assistance in keeping you accountable. Let them know what triggers you find most challenging and discuss strategies to overcome them together. By involving your partner in your quitting journey, you not only strengthen your bond but also create a sense of shared responsibility in protecting your unborn child.

In addition to seeking support from your loved ones, joining a support group can provide immense benefits. Support groups are made up of individuals who are going through a similar experience as you – quitting smoking while being pregnant. These groups offer a safe and non-judgmental space to share your thoughts, struggles, and successes. The empathy and encouragement you receive from fellow group members can be incredibly motivating and help you stay on track.

Accountability is another key element in successfully quitting smoking during pregnancy. Holding yourself accountable means having a strong commitment and staying true to your decision to quit. But we all know that cravings and withdrawal symptoms can be incredibly challenging, especially during the early stages of quitting. This is where establishing a system of accountability can make all the difference.

One effective way to stay accountable is by setting goals and tracking your progress. Start by setting a quit date and mark it on your calendar, symbolizing the beginning of your smoke-free journey. From there, set milestones for yourself – perhaps a week without smoking, then a month, and so on. These milestones act as mini-celebrations, rewarding your progress and motivating you to keep going.

Tracking your progress can be done in various ways. Some find it helpful to keep a journal, documenting their cravings, triggers, and feelings throughout the quitting process. Others prefer using smartphone apps specifically designed to track smoking cessation progress. These apps can offer daily tips, motivational messages, and even financial calculations to show you the amount of money you have saved by not smoking. Choose the method that resonates with you the most and make it a routine part of your journey.

While supportive communication and accountability are crucial in managing cravings and withdrawal symptoms, it is essential to remember that quitting smoking during pregnancy is a personal decision motivated by the health and well-being of your unborn baby. It is normal to face challenges and setbacks along the way, but it is important to stay focused on your ultimate goal and not let them discourage you.

Celebrating Success and Staying Resilient

Quitting smoking is no easy feat, especially during pregnancy when hormones are fluctuating and emotions are heightened. It requires a great deal of resilience to resist the urge to light up, especially when faced with challenging situations or triggers. However, with the right mindset and tools, you can conquer this journey and protect your baby's health. In this section, we will provide you with tips on self-reward, self-reflection, and maintaining a positive outlook in the face of challenges.

Self-Reward:

Rewarding yourself for each accomplishment is an essential part of the quitting process. It acknowledges your efforts and serves as a reminder that your hard work is paying off. When you successfully resist the temptation to smoke, treat yourself to something you enjoy. It could be a small indulgence like a bubble bath, a new book, or a piece of your favourite dessert. The key is to choose rewards that align with your personal preferences and bring you joy. By doing so, you create positive associations with the act of quitting and reinforce your determination to stay smoke-free.

Another effective way to reward yourself is by setting up a rewards system. For instance, for every week or month you remain smoke-free, allocate a certain amount of money towards a larger reward, such as a spa day or a weekend getaway. This not only gives you something to look forward to but also serves as a tangible reminder of your progress and the benefits of quitting. Celebrating success milestones in this way can help you stay motivated and provide a sense of accomplishment in your journey towards a smoke-free pregnancy.

Self-Reflection:

Self-reflection is an important aspect of the quitting process. It allows you to gain a deeper understanding of your smoking habits, triggers, and coping mechanisms. By analysing your patterns and behaviours, you can identify potential pitfalls and develop strategies to overcome them. Taking the time to reflect on your journey will enable you to make conscious choices and break free from the cycle of smoking.

To engage in self-reflection, start by keeping a journal. Document your cravings, emotions, and triggers throughout the day. By doing so, you will start to notice patterns and trends. For example, you may find that you are more likely to crave a cigarette when you feel stressed or anxious. Armed with this knowledge, you can proactively find alternative ways to manage stress, such as deep breathing exercises, meditation, or engaging in a soothing activity like knitting or painting.

In addition to journaling, seeking support from others who have successfully quit smoking during pregnancy can be invaluable. Joining a support group or online forum can provide a sense of community, share experiences, and provide encouragement. Hearing stories of triumph from others who have overcome similar challenges can be highly motivating and inspire you to stay on track. Remember, you are not alone on this journey; there are countless others who have faced similar obstacles and emerged victorious.

Maintaining a Positive Outlook:

Maintaining a positive outlook is crucial when quitting smoking during pregnancy. It is natural to experience ups and downs along the way, but it is your mindset that can make all the difference. A positive attitude will not only help you stay resilient but also enable you to navigate challenges more effectively.

One effective technique for maintaining a positive
mindset is to focus on the benefits of quitting
smoking, both for yourself and your baby. Remind
yourself of the countless health benefits, such as
improved oxygen flow to the baby, reduced risk of
complications, and increased chances of a healthy
birth weight. Visualize your baby growing strong and
healthy in a smoke-free environment. This
visualization exercise can be a powerful tool in
reinforcing your commitment and reminding you of
the bigger picture.

Another helpful strategy is to replace negative
thoughts with positive affirmations. Repeat
affirmations such as "I am strong," "I am capable,"
and "I am a non-smoker" as a way to reprogram your
mindset and strengthen your resolve. Surround
yourself with positive influences, whether it is
uplifting music, inspirational books, or motivational
quotes. These small but consistent efforts can make a
significant impact on your overall outlook and
contribute to your success in quitting smoking during
pregnancy.

Chapter 6: Nurturing a Healthy Pregnancy

Proper Nutrition for a Smoke-Free Pregnancy

When you make the decision to quit smoking during pregnancy, you have already taken a monumental step towards safeguarding the health and well-being of both you and your baby. However, it is important to note that smoking cessation alone is not enough. Adopting a healthy diet that meets your nutritional needs is imperative to ensure proper foetal development and to mitigate any potential risks associated with smoking.

1. Why is proper nutrition important during pregnancy after quitting smoking?

Quitting smoking is undoubtedly beneficial for your health and the health of your baby. However, smoking depletes the body of essential nutrients, and simply quitting may not be enough to replenish what has been lost. Proper nutrition plays a vital role in supporting foetal growth, reducing the risk of complications, and maintaining your own well-being during pregnancy and beyond.

2. Dietary recommendations for a smoke-free pregnancy:

When it comes to nutrition during pregnancy, it is important to follow a well-balanced and varied diet that includes all the necessary nutrients. Here are some dietary recommendations to consider:

a. Increase your intake of fruits and vegetables: Fruits and vegetables are rich in essential vitamins and minerals and provide important antioxidants that can help protect against cellular damage caused by smoking. Aim to include a variety of colourful fruits and vegetables in your meals and snacks to ensure you receive a wide range of nutrients.

b. Choose whole grains: Whole grains such as brown rice, whole wheat bread, and quinoa are rich in fibre and provide important nutrients like B vitamins and iron. They can also help regulate blood sugar levels and promote healthy digestion.

c. Include lean proteins: Protein is essential for foetal growth and development. opt for lean sources of protein such as lean meats, poultry, fish, eggs, legumes, and tofu. These protein-rich foods are also rich in other important nutrients like iron and omega-3 fatty acids.

d. Incorporate healthy fats: Fats are an important part of a healthy diet and play a crucial role in foetal brain development. Include foods rich in omega-3 fatty acids like fatty fish (salmon, sardines), walnuts, chia seeds, and flaxseeds. However, it is important to consume these fats in moderation, as they are high in calories.

e. Stay hydrated: Staying hydrated is crucial for both you and your baby. Aim to drink at least 8-10 glasses of water per day and avoid sugary drinks. Opt for water, herbal teas, and natural fruit juices instead.

3. Essential nutrients for a smoke-free pregnancy:

a. Folate: Folate is a B vitamin that plays a crucial role in foetal development, particularly in preventing neural tube defects. Smoking has been shown to deplete folate levels in the body, so it is important to ensure adequate intake during pregnancy. Good sources of folate include leafy green vegetables, citrus fruits, legumes, and fortified cereals.

b. Iron: Iron is essential for the production of red blood cells and the delivery of oxygen to both you and your baby. Smoking can deplete iron levels in the body, so it is important to incorporate iron-rich foods like lean meats, poultry, fish, legumes, and fortified cereals into your diet. Pairing iron-rich foods with Vitamin C-rich foods can enhance iron absorption.

c. Vitamin C: Vitamin C is an important antioxidant that helps protect against cellular damage caused by smoking. Good sources of Vitamin C include citrus fruits, berries, kiwi, bell peppers, and broccoli.

d. Calcium: Calcium is essential for the development of strong bones and teeth in both you and your baby. It also plays a role in nerve function and muscle contraction. Good sources of calcium include milk, yogurt, cheese, tofu, almonds, and leafy green vegetables.

e. Omega-3 fatty acids: Omega-3 fatty acids, particularly DHA, are crucial for foetal brain development. Smoking has been shown to negatively impact DHA levels in the body, so it is important to include foods rich in omega-3 fatty acids in your diet. This includes fatty fish like salmon and sardines, walnuts, chia seeds, and flaxseeds.

4. The role of a balanced diet in supporting foetal development:

A balanced diet during pregnancy is crucial for supporting proper foetal development. By providing your body with essential nutrients through a variety of wholesome foods, you are ensuring that your baby receives the necessary building blocks for growth and development.

A balanced diet not only supports the physical needs of your baby but also contributes to their cognitive and emotional development. It can help reduce the risk of complications during pregnancy, such as gestational diabetes and preeclampsia, both of which can be exacerbated by smoking.

It is important to remember that a balanced diet alone cannot completely mitigate the potential risks associated with smoking during pregnancy. However, by combining a healthy diet with smoking cessation, you are taking significant steps towards ensuring the best possible outcomes for both you and your baby.

Regular Exercise and Physical Well-being

Exercise is often overlooked during pregnancy, with many women feeling apprehensive or unsure about what they can and cannot do. However, maintaining regular physical activity during this crucial time brings numerous benefits that can greatly contribute to the well-being of both mother and baby.

Firstly, regular exercise during pregnancy can help improve overall fitness levels. Staying active helps maintain a healthy weight, reduces the risk of gestational diabetes, and promotes cardiovascular health. It also strengthens muscles, increasing endurance and flexibility, which can be particularly beneficial during labor and delivery.

Engaging in moderate-intensity activities such as brisk walking, swimming, and prenatal yoga can elevate heart rate and circulation without causing excess strain on the body. It is important to note that exercising during pregnancy does not aim for weight loss or intense muscle building; instead, it focuses on maintaining a healthy body and mind.

Alongside physical benefits, exercise during pregnancy offers remarkable psychological rewards. Pregnancy brings about changes in a woman's body and emotions, which can sometimes lead to feelings of anxiety, stress, and low mood. By incorporating regular exercise into their routine, pregnant women can alleviate these negative emotions and promote a more positive mindset.

Exercise releases endorphins, also known as the "feel-good" hormones, which act as natural mood enhancers. These endorphins help reduce stress, improve sleep patterns, and boost overall mental well-being. Engaging in physical activity also provides a healthy distraction from the challenges and discomforts that can accompany pregnancy, allowing women to focus on their body's strength and the incredible journey they are undertaking.

Maintaining a regular exercise routine can also contribute to a healthier pregnancy by reducing the risk of complications. Gestational diabetes, high blood pressure, and preeclampsia are all conditions that can arise during pregnancy and pose risks to both the mother and the baby. However, studies have shown that regular exercise can significantly reduce the chances of developing these conditions.

Research conducted by the American College of Obstetricians and Gynaecologists (ACOG) has found that exercising during pregnancy can lower the risk of gestational diabetes by nearly 30%. Similarly, a study published in the British Journal of Sports Medicine reported a 35% lower risk of preeclampsia among women who engaged in regular physical activity.

The benefits of exercise during pregnancy are not limited to the mother alone. The growing foetus also reaps the advantages of maternal physical activity. Regular exercise helps improve placental blood flow, which in turn increases oxygen and nutrient supply to the baby. This enhanced blood flow contributes to the development of a healthier placenta, supporting optimal growth and development of the foetus.

Furthermore, exercise has been found to have a positive impact on the baby's cognitive development. Research conducted at the University of Montreal found that babies born to women who exercised during pregnancy exhibited enhanced brain function compared to those born to mothers who were less physically active. Exercise has also been shown to reduce the risk of neural tube defects and promote better birth outcomes.

While exercise during pregnancy is generally considered safe and beneficial, it is essential to consult with a healthcare provider before embarking on any exercise regimen. Medical professionals can provide guidance based on individual circumstances and recommend appropriate exercises based on the overall health of the mother and the baby.

When starting an exercise routine during pregnancy, it is important to begin slowly and gradually increase intensity and duration. Warm-up exercises, such as stretching and gentle movements, are crucial to prepare the body for physical activity and reduce the risk of injury. Additionally, wearing comfortable, supportive footwear and loose-fitting clothing is vital to ensure optimal comfort during exercise.

Modifying exercises as the pregnancy progresses is necessary to accommodate the changing needs of the body. As the baby grows and the centre of gravity shifts, certain activities may become more challenging. For example, exercises that involve lying flat on the back are generally not recommended beyond the first trimester as they can restrict blood flow to the uterus.

Sufficient hydration is also essential during exercise to prevent dehydration and ensure the well-being of both mother and baby. It is recommended to drink water before, during, and after physical activity, particularly in hot and humid conditions.

Incorporating regular physical activity into a daily routine during pregnancy may require some adjustments and time management. However, the benefits far outweigh the challenges. Engaging in activities such as prenatal yoga classes, swimming, and even simply going for a walk can be enjoyable ways to stay active and promote a healthy pregnancy.

Notably, exercising during pregnancy is not advised in certain circumstances. If a pregnant woman has any medical complications, such as placenta previa, preterm labor, or a history of miscarriage, it may be necessary to avoid or modify physical activity. Consulting with a healthcare provider is crucial for personalized and appropriate advice.

Mental and Emotional Well-being

Stress management is a crucial aspect of maintaining mental and emotional well-being. Pregnancy itself can be stressful, and quitting smoking can add an extra layer of anxiety and tension. Finding healthy ways to cope with stress is essential for both you and your baby. One effective technique is deep breathing exercises. Taking slow, deep breaths can help calm your mind and relax your body. Close your eyes, focus on your breathing, and let go of any tension with every exhale. Another helpful strategy is practicing mindfulness. Mindfulness involves being fully present and engaged in the moment, without judgment. This can be done through activities such as meditation, yoga, or simply taking a peaceful walk-in nature. These practices can help reduce stress levels and promote a sense of mental tranquillity.

Managing your mental and emotional well-being during pregnancy after quitting smoking is a continuous process. It requires dedication, self-reflection, and patience with yourself. Remember to be kind to yourself and give yourself grace. This is a transformative journey, and it is natural to experience ups and downs. Embrace the journey and allow yourself to grow and evolve, not just as a non-smoker, but also as a person.

Regular Prenatal Care and Medical Check-ups

When a woman becomes pregnant, her body undergoes numerous changes to accommodate the growing life within her. These changes not only impact her physically but also give rise to a range of emotions, questions, and concerns. Regular prenatal care provides a platform for expectant mothers to address these concerns, receive guidance, and stay informed about the progress of their pregnancy.

One of the primary reasons why regular prenatal care visits are so important is to monitor foetal growth. By tracking the growth of the baby, healthcare providers can ensure that the baby is developing properly and identify any potential deviations from the norm. This is especially critical for pregnant women who have quit smoking, as smoking during pregnancy can lead to various complications and growth-related issues for the baby.

During these visits, healthcare providers may conduct a variety of tests and examinations to assess the well-being of both the mother and the baby. Tests such as ultrasounds, blood pressure measurements, and blood tests, among others, help monitor the overall health of the pregnant woman and detect any potential complications. These tests also enable healthcare providers to track the baby's growth, assess the development of vital organs, and identify any potential anomalies early on.

In addition to monitoring foetal growth, regular prenatal care visits also provide an opportunity to address any potential complications that may arise during pregnancy. Pregnancy can bring about a whole host of health concerns, ranging from gestational diabetes and preeclampsia to preterm labor and miscarriage. While quitting smoking is a significant step towards ensuring a healthy pregnancy, it does not eliminate the possibility of other complications.

During prenatal care visits, healthcare providers can assess the mother's risk factors and identify any preexisting conditions that may require special attention. They can also offer guidance on managing these conditions and provide necessary treatments to mitigate potential risks. Regular check-ups allow healthcare providers to closely monitor the progress of the pregnancy and intervene if any complications arise, thus ensuring the best possible outcome for both the mother and the baby.

Moreover, regular prenatal care visits serve as a valuable source of information and education for expectant mothers. Pregnancy is a journey filled with endless questions and uncertainties. By attending these visits, pregnant women can gain access to a vast array of resources and support systems that can provide them with the knowledge and tools they need to make informed decisions about their health and the health of their baby.

Additionally, healthcare providers can offer guidance on various aspects of pregnancy, such as healthy eating, exercise, and stress management. They can provide information about the potential risks of smoking during pregnancy, reinforcing the decision to quit and offering further motivation to stay smoke-free. Regular check-ups provide an ideal forum for pregnant women to seek guidance, discuss any concerns, and receive personalized advice tailored to their specific needs and circumstances.

I believe that with proper care, support, and guidance, pregnant women who have quit smoking can successfully navigate their journey to motherhood, and provide their babies with a healthy start in life. I hope that this guide serves as a valuable resource for you, empowering to take control of your health and protect your baby. Remember, you have the power to make a positive and lasting impact on your baby's future.

Celebrating a Smoke-Free Pregnancy

The decision to quit smoking during pregnancy is undoubtedly a challenging one. I understand that as someone who has witnessed the struggles and triumphs of numerous women trying to quit. But it is also a decision that deserves immense celebration. When a pregnant woman commits to a smoke-free journey, she is not only taking a significant step towards the well-being of her baby but also towards her own health.

I have had the privilege of working with pregnant women who have successfully quit smoking, and each journey has been an inspiration. Take the case of Sarah, a determined woman who made the decision to quit smoking as soon as she found out she was pregnant. Sarah had been a smoker for almost a decade and had tried quitting multiple times before without success. However, the moment she discovered that she was carrying a tiny, fragile life within her, everything changed.

For Sarah, quitting smoking was not just about herself anymore; it was about the health and well-being of her baby. She sought guidance, support, and resources to help her through the difficult process. With the help of her healthcare provider and the support of her family and friends, Sarah embarked on a smoke-free journey that would forever change her life.

As the weeks went by, Sarah noticed significant improvements in her health. Her energy levels increased, and she no longer experienced the shortness of breath that had become a constant companion during her smoking days. The positive changes she experienced motivated her to stay strong in her resolve to remain smoke-free. And most importantly, she knew she was giving her baby the best possible start in life.

Sarah's story exemplifies the triumph that can be achieved through determination, support, and the will to protect one's unborn child. It is stories like this that continue to inspire and encourage pregnant women who are on the same journey.

Research has consistently shown that quitting smoking during pregnancy has numerous benefits for both the mother and baby. One study conducted at the University of Melbourne found that the risk of preterm birth significantly decreased among pregnant women who quit smoking compared to those who continued to smoke. Another study published in the Journal of the American Medical Association revealed that quitting smoking during pregnancy reduced the chances of stillbirth and sudden infant death syndrome (SIDS).

Quitting smoking during pregnancy also improves the overall oxygen supply to the developing foetus, ensuring healthier growth and development. It helps prevent complications such as low birth weight and placental problems that can have long-term effects on the baby. Additionally, it reduces the risk of respiratory problems and asthma in children.

But the benefits of a smoke-free pregnancy go beyond physical health. It also has a positive impact on mental and emotional well-being. Quitting smoking can increase feelings of empowerment and self-confidence, giving women a sense of control over their own health and the health of their baby. It creates an environment of positivity and hope, fostering a strong bond between mother and child.

While the decision to quit smoking during pregnancy is commendable, it is essential to acknowledge that it can be a challenging journey. Nicotine addiction is a powerful force, and the withdrawal symptoms can be difficult to manage. That is why support and resources are crucial in ensuring a successful quit attempt.

Healthcare providers play a vital role in this journey by offering guidance, tools, and evidence-based strategies to help pregnant women quit smoking. They can provide information about the available nicotine replacement therapies that are safe during pregnancy, such as nicotine patches or gum. They can also connect pregnant women with support groups or counselling services that offer emotional support and practical advice.

In addition to professional support, having a strong support system at home is equally important. Family members, friends, and partners can provide encouragement and hold pregnant women accountable, creating a smoke-free environment that is conducive to their success. Celebrating each milestone achieved, no matter how small, can provide the motivation needed to continue along the smoke-free journey.

Remember, celebrating a smoke-free pregnancy is not just about the absence of smoking. It is about embracing a healthier lifestyle, making choices that benefit both the mother and baby. Engaging in regular exercise, eating a well-balanced diet, and practicing relaxation techniques can all contribute to a healthier pregnancy.

Chapter 7: Staying Smoke-Free After Pregnancy

Balancing the responsibilities of motherhood and maintaining a smoke-free lifestyle requires dedication, support, and a strong sense of commitment. It is important to remember that every woman's journey is unique, and what works for one may not work for another. That being said, here are some useful tips that helped me navigate this path:

1. Educate Yourself: Knowledge is power. Understanding the risks associated with smoking during pregnancy can serve as a powerful motivator to quit. Learn about the harm that tobacco smoke can cause to the baby's development and how it can increase the risk of premature birth, low birth weight, and other complications.

2. Find Support: Surround yourself with people who support your decision to quit smoking. Seek the support of your partner, family, and friends. Their encouragement and understanding will play a crucial role in your journey towards a smoke-free life. Additionally, consider joining support groups or online communities where you can connect with other women going through a similar experience. Sharing your challenges and triumphs with others can be immensely empowering.

3. Seek Professional Help: There is a wide range of resources available to help you quit smoking during pregnancy. Speak to your healthcare provider and ask for guidance. They may recommend nicotine replacement therapy or prescribe medications to aid in your quitting journey. Their expertise and support can make a significant difference in your success.

4. Develop Healthy Coping Mechanisms: Quitting smoking can be challenging, especially during times of stress. It is important to develop healthy coping mechanisms that can replace the urge to smoke. Engage in activities that bring you joy, such as gentle

exercise, meditation, or creative hobbies. Surround yourself with positive distractions, and remember that you are not alone in this journey.

5. Practice Self-Care: Motherhood can be overwhelming, and it is important to prioritize your own well-being. Take time for yourself, indulge in activities that relax and rejuvenate you. Engage in self-care practices such as taking a warm bath, reading a book, or spending quality time with loved ones. By taking care of yourself, you can better care for your baby.

6. Focus on the Bond with Your Baby: Embrace the wonders of motherhood and cherish the bond you share with your baby. Every decision you make to maintain a smoke-free lifestyle is an act of love for your child. Visualize the healthy and smoke-free future that awaits your baby, and let that vision guide you through the challenges you may encounter.

Creating a Supportive Postpartum Environment

After finally overcoming the challenges of smoking during pregnancy and successfully giving birth to a healthy baby, the journey towards a smoke-free life continues. The postpartum period is a critical phase that requires utmost care, attention, and support. It is during this time that new mothers may face numerous emotional and physical changes, making them vulnerable to relapse. Without the right support system in place, the risk of reverting back to old habits becomes increasingly likely.

Managing stress is crucial during the postpartum period. The demands of caring for a newborn, combined with other stressors such as hormonal changes, lack of sleep, and adjusting to new routines, can overwhelm new mothers. It is essential to recognize that stress can be a trigger for relapse and take proactive steps to manage it effectively.

One effective strategy to manage stress is to set realistic expectations. As a new mother, it is natural to feel the pressure to be a perfect parent. However, it is important to remember that being a good parent does not mean being flawless. It is okay to ask for help and delegate tasks when necessary. Creating a support network with family and friends who can assist with household chores, childcare, and emotional support can make a world of difference. This not only provides new mothers with the opportunity to rest and recharge but also reduces the likelihood of turning to smoking as a coping mechanism.

Self-care is another vital aspect of managing stress. Taking the time to engage in activities that bring joy and relaxation can significantly impact a new mother's emotional well-being. This can include practicing mindfulness or meditation, indulging in a hobby, or simply having a peaceful moment alone. By prioritizing self-care, new mothers can better cope with stress and reduce the urge to rely on smoking as a means of escape.

Seeking help when needed is crucial for maintaining a smoke-free postpartum period. It is important to remember that reaching out for support is a sign of strength, not weakness. Whether it is discussing challenges faced with a healthcare provider, attending support groups, or seeking therapy, there are various resources available to help new mothers navigate this delicate phase.

Healthcare providers play a pivotal role in supporting new mothers on their smoke-free journey. They can provide guidance, offer resources, and monitor the progress made. Regular check-ups offer an opportunity to discuss any concerns, receive encouragement, and address any triggers that may be present, minimizing the risk of relapse.

In addition to professional help, connecting with other new mothers who are also on a smoke-free journey can be immensely beneficial. Online communities, support groups, or even friends who have gone through a similar experience can provide a safe space to share struggles, celebrate victories, and gain inspiration. By surrounding yourself with individuals who understand the challenges faced and offer support, the journey towards a smoke-free postpartum becomes less daunting.

Communication plays a vital role in creating a supportive postpartum environment. Openly discussing thoughts, fears, and challenges with loved ones can foster understanding and empathy. Loved ones, such as partners, family members, and close friends, can provide emotional support, encouragement, and lend a helping hand when needed. By involving them in the journey, new mothers can feel less isolated and more motivated to stay smoke-free.

Setting boundaries is an essential part of effective communication. It is important to clearly communicate your expectations and needs to loved ones. This may involve politely asking them not to smoke around you or your baby, requesting their understanding and support, and explaining the importance of a smoke-free environment for the health and well-being of all involved. By setting boundaries and communicating them effectively, new mothers can establish a supportive and smoke-free atmosphere for themselves and their babies.

It is also crucial to address any potential triggers that may arise in the postpartum period. Certain situations or environments, such as social gatherings where others may be smoking, can present challenges. By discussing these triggers with loved ones, they can become allies in finding solutions and creating alternative strategies to cope with situations that may arise. For example, if attending a social event where smoking is likely, a loved one can provide extra support by being present, engaging in conversation, or distracting the new mother from the urge to smoke.

Lastly, but certainly not least, it is important for new mothers to celebrate their accomplishments and milestones along the way. Each smoke-free day is a triumph to be acknowledged and celebrated. By recognizing and celebrating progress, new mothers can build self-confidence and reinforce their commitment to maintaining a smoke-free lifestyle.

Healthy Coping Mechanisms and Stress Reduction

Self-Care Practices:

One of the most important aspects of stress reduction is taking care of yourself. Often, as mothers, we tend to put the needs of our baby before our own. However, it is crucial to remember that you cannot pour from an empty cup. By prioritizing self-care, you can better fulfil your role as a mother and protect your own mental health.

There are many self-care practices you can incorporate into your daily routine. These can include simple activities such as taking a warm bath, treating yourself to a cup of herbal tea, or indulging in your favourite hobby. Remember, self-care looks different for everyone, so find activities that bring you joy and make you feel refreshed and rejuvenated.

Time Management:

Time management is another important aspect of reducing stress. As a new mother, your days may feel chaotic and filled with endless tasks. By implementing effective time management techniques, you can regain a sense of control and reduce the feeling of overwhelm.

Start by creating a daily schedule or to-do list. Prioritize your tasks, allowing for flexibility as unexpected events may arise. Break your tasks into smaller, more manageable steps, as this can help you feel a sense of accomplishment as you tick things off your list. Remember to allocate time for self-care activities, ensuring that you are taking care of yourself amidst your daily responsibilities.

Engaging in Relaxation Activities:

Engaging in activities that promote relaxation and well-being is crucial in reducing stress. Here are a few relaxation techniques that you can incorporate into your routine:

1. Deep Breathing Exercises:

Deep breathing exercises are a powerful tool for stress reduction. Find a quiet place where you can sit comfortably. Close your eyes and take slow, deep breaths, inhaling through your nose and exhaling through your mouth. Focus on your breath, allowing it to bring you a sense of calm and relaxation. Practice deep breathing exercises whenever you feel overwhelmed or stressed.

2. Meditation:

Meditation is a practice that can help quiet the mind and reduce stress. Find a comfortable position and close your eyes. Focus on your breath or choose a specific mantra or visualization to guide your meditation. Allow your thoughts to come and go without judgment, returning your focus to your breath or chosen point of focus. Even a few minutes of meditation each day can help you find a sense of inner peace and reduce stress.

3. Gentle Exercise or Yoga:

Engaging in gentle exercise or yoga can also help reduce stress and promote relaxation. Physical activity releases endorphins, which are known as the feel-good hormones. These hormones can help elevate your mood and reduce stress levels. Choose exercises that are safe and suitable for your post-pregnancy body and consult with your healthcare provider before starting any new exercise regime.

4. Journaling:

Writing in a journal can be a therapeutic way to process your thoughts and emotions, reducing stress in the process. Take a few minutes each day to write down your thoughts, feelings, and any stressors you may be experiencing. This practice can help clear your mind and provide a sense of relief, allowing you to better manage stress.

Setting a Positive Example for the Child

Smoking during pregnancy is not only harmful to your own health but also puts the health of your baby at risk. Research has shown that smoking while pregnant increases the risk of premature birth, low birth weight, and developmental issues. Babies born to mothers who smoke are more likely to have respiratory problems, such as asthma and bronchitis, and are at a higher risk for sudden infant death syndrome (SIDS). These risks alone should be enough to motivate any expectant mother to quit smoking.

But let's delve deeper into the concept of setting a positive example for your child. By choosing to go smoke-free during your pregnancy and beyond, you are not only protecting your child's physical health but also sending a powerful message about healthy habits and self-care.

Children learn by observing and imitating their parents. They look up to us as role models, absorbing our behaviours and attitudes like sponges. When you make the commitment to quit smoking, you are showing your child that their health and well-being are a top priority for you. You are demonstrating the importance of making choices that promote a healthy and smoke-free lifestyle.

As your child grows older, they will encounter various influences, both positive and negative, that may shape their attitudes towards smoking. By maintaining a smoke-free environment and openly discussing the dangers of smoking, you empower your child to make informed decisions and resist peer pressure. They will understand from a young age that smoking is harmful, addictive, and not something they should engage in.

Studies have shown that children whose parents smoke are more likely to smoke themselves when they reach adolescence. By setting a positive example and actively promoting a smoke-free household, you significantly reduce the likelihood of your child becoming a smoker. You are instilling in them the values of self-respect, responsibility, and a commitment to a healthy lifestyle.

Furthermore, quitting smoking during pregnancy and continuing to lead a smoke-free life after your baby is born is a powerful way to protect their overall development. Research has shown that exposure to second-hand smoke can have detrimental effects on a child's cognitive and behavioral development. It can lead to learning difficulties, attention deficit disorders, and behavioral problems. By ensuring a smoke-free environment, you are providing your child with the best chance for a healthy and balanced upbringing.

Start by creating a smoke-free home. Remove all smoking paraphernalia, such as ashtrays and lighters, and clean your house thoroughly to eliminate any residual smoke, Odor. This will not only make it easier for you to resist temptation but also create a healthier and welcoming environment for your child.

Chapter 8: Additional Resources and Support

Online Communities and Support Groups

When I first started my research on online communities and support groups for pregnant women quitting smoking, I was amazed by the wealth of resources available. From dedicated websites to social media groups, there are numerous platforms that cater to this specific group of individuals. These communities offer a safe and supportive space where women can connect with others who share their journey, understand their struggles, and celebrate their achievements.

One of the major benefits of joining an online community or support group for pregnant women is the opportunity to connect with others who are going through similar experiences. Quitting smoking is not an easy task, especially during pregnancy when hormones can intensify cravings and withdrawal symptoms. Having the support of individuals who understand these struggles can make a world of difference. Whether it is seeking advice on how to cope with cravings or finding motivation to stay smoke-free, knowing that there are others who can relate and offer support can be incredibly empowering.

Furthermore, these online communities and support groups foster a sense of belonging and provide a judgment-free zone. Many women who smoke during pregnancy face stigma and judgment from society. However, in these virtual spaces, they can freely discuss their challenges without the fear of being shamed or criticized. This safe environment allows women to be open and honest about their struggles and seek guidance from a community that understands the complexities of quitting smoking during pregnancy.

Aside from emotional support, these online communities and support groups also provide valuable information and resources. Pregnant women can benefit from shared experiences and learn about various strategies and tools for quitting smoking. Whether it is through success stories, tips for managing cravings, or recommendations for alternative coping mechanisms, these communities are a treasure trove of knowledge and support. By actively participating in discussions and engaging with other members, women can gain valuable insights and strategies to help them on their smoke-free journey.

Success stories play a crucial role in motivating and inspiring individuals to quit smoking. Hearing about others' accomplishments can instil a sense of hope and belief in one's ability to quit. Online communities and support groups often have designated sections where women can share their success stories. These stories serve as a source of inspiration and encouragement, reminding women that quitting smoking is indeed possible. Reading about the triumphs and transformations of others who have walked the same path can be incredibly uplifting and motivating.

In addition to emotional support and information sharing, some online communities and support groups also offer structured programs or activities that can further aid in smoking cessation. These programs may include weekly challenges, goal setting exercises, or even live video sessions with healthcare professionals specializing in smoking cessation. By participating in such programs, women can receive expert guidance and actively work towards their goal of quitting smoking.

It is important to note that while online communities and support groups for pregnant women quitting smoking can be immensely helpful, they should not replace professional medical advice. It is crucial for women to consult with their healthcare providers to develop a personalized quit plan and ensure their safety and the safety of their baby throughout the quitting process. The online communities and support groups should be viewed as a supplemental resource, providing support and guidance in conjunction with medical advice.

As with any online community or support group, it is essential to choose a platform that is reputable and trustworthy. Take the time to research different platforms, read reviews, and understand the rules and guidelines of each community. Look for platforms that prioritize privacy and security, as well as those that create a positive and supportive atmosphere. Engage in discussions, ask questions, and introduce yourself to the community. The more involved you are, the more you will benefit from the wealth of knowledge and support available.

Helplines and Hotlines

1. National Quitline:

The National Quitline is a government-funded helpline specifically designed to help individuals quit smoking. They have trained counsellors available 24/7 to provide support and information. The counsellors can guide women on effective cessation methods, address concerns, and provide motivation to overcome the challenges of quitting smoking during pregnancy. Some Quitline's also offer free nicotine replacement therapy (NRT) products to eligible individuals.

Contact Information:

- National Quitline: 1-800-QUIT-NOW

- Website: www.smokefree.gov

2. American Lung Association:

The American Lung Association offers a dedicated helpline for pregnant women who want to quit smoking and protect their baby's health. The helpline connects callers with experienced tobacco cessation counsellors who can provide guidance and support tailored specifically for pregnant women. Whether it is about managing withdrawal symptoms, finding alternative coping strategies, or addressing relapse triggers, these counsellors are equipped with the necessary knowledge to help women through the process.

Contact Information:

- American Lung Association Helpline: 1-800-LUNGUSA

- Website: www.lung.org

3. March of Dimes:

The March of Dimes provides a helpline for pregnant women looking for assistance in quitting smoking. Their knowledgeable staff members can offer guidance on creating a personalized quit plan, coping with cravings and urges, managing stress, and seeking additional resources when needed. The March of Dimes helpline also educates women about the risks of smoking during pregnancy and highlights the positive impact of quitting on the health of the baby.

Contact Information:

- March of Dimes Pregnancy and Newborn Helpline: 1-888-588-3433

- Website: www.marchofdimes.org

4. Baby & Me – Tobacco Free Program:

The Baby & Me – Tobacco Free Program is a unique initiative that offers counselling and support to pregnant women who want to quit smoking. This program also goes a step further by providing incentives to encourage and reward women for their successful cessation. By participating in the program, women receive support from trained professionals, engage in group counselling sessions, and have access to educational materials that promote a smoke-free lifestyle during and after pregnancy.

Contact Information:

- Baby & Me – Tobacco Free Program: 1-800-TRY-TO-STOP

- Website: www.babyandmetobaccofree.org

5. National Smokers' Quitline:

The National Smokers' Quitline is another helpline that offers support to pregnant women who are trying to quit smoking. Their trained counsellors provide non-judgmental assistance to women, helping them overcome the challenges associated with quitting. The helpline offers resources such as an online community, information on medication options, and strategies to cope with cravings and triggers.

Contact Information:

- National Smokers' Quitline: 1-800-784-8669

- Website: www.smokefree.gov

6. Your Healthcare Provider:

Apart from helplines and hotlines, pregnant women can also reach out to their healthcare provider for support and guidance in quitting smoking. Healthcare professionals, including doctors, nurses, and midwives, have a wealth of knowledge about smoking cessation, the effects of smoking on pregnancy, and the available resources to help women combat this addiction. They can offer personalized advice, recommend cessation methods, and monitor the progress of the quitting journey.

Contact Information:

- Schedule an appointment with your healthcare provider to discuss smoking cessation options.

It's important to note that the above-listed helplines and hotlines are just a starting point for pregnant women seeking support in quitting smoking. Other local organizations and resources may also be available, depending on the area in which you reside. One should explore community health centres, local Department of Health websites, and pregnancy support groups to discover additional assistance options suitable for one's specific needs and preferences.

Make sure to note the operating hours of each helpline and hotline for quick reference. While some helplines operate 24/7, others have specific hours of operation. It's essential to know when assistance is readily available.

Finally, the services provided by each helpline may differ slightly. Some may focus primarily on counselling and providing emotional support, while others may also offer educational materials, cessation medication guidance, or connections to local support groups. Pregnant women should reach out to multiple helplines to find the one that aligns best with their needs and preferences.

Remember, quitting smoking is a challenging journey, especially during pregnancy. However, with the support and guidance offered by helplines and hotlines, pregnant women can find the strength and resources they need to protect the health of their baby. Reach out, make that call, and stay committed to the goal of providing a smoke-free environment for both you and your child.

Recommended Books and Resources

1. "The Pregnancy Planner & Journal: A Week-by-Week Guide to a Healthy Pregnancy" by Lisa Trumbauer:

This comprehensive guide offers expectant mothers a week-by-week overview of their pregnancy journey. While it does not focus solely on smoking cessation, it provides valuable information about foetal development, common pregnancy concerns, and maintaining a healthy lifestyle during pregnancy. By understanding how smoking can impact our growing baby, we can gain motivation and determination to quit for good.

2. "The New Pregnancy and Childbirth: Choices and Challenges" by Sheila Kitzinger:

While this book delves into various aspects of pregnancy and childbirth, it also addresses the challenges faced by women trying to quit smoking during pregnancy. It provides insights into the effects of smoking on the baby's health and offers strategies to overcome addiction. The book emphasizes the importance of seeking support from professionals and loved ones during this challenging journey.

3. "Easy way for Mothers: A Guide to Quitting Smoking" by Allen Carr:

Allen Carr's Easy way method has gained widespread acclaim for helping individuals quit smoking permanently. This book specifically caters to expectant mothers, guiding them through the process of quitting without the use of willpower or substitutes. It offers practical advice, real-life stories, and techniques that address the unique challenges faced by pregnant women. By adopting the Easy way method, we can break free from the grip of nicotine addiction and ensure a healthier future for our babies.

4. "Smoking Cessation During Pregnancy: A Clinician's Guide to Helping Pregnant Women Quit Smoking" by Tina Grossman-Clarke and Kimber Richter:

Written by renowned experts in the field, this book offers a comprehensive guide for healthcare professionals working with pregnant women who smoke. Although it is primarily aimed at clinicians, it can prove immensely beneficial for expectant mothers seeking to understand the various strategies and interventions that can aid in smoking cessation. By familiarizing ourselves with the perspectives and recommendations of healthcare professionals, we can actively engage in discussions with our own caregivers and make informed decisions.

5. "Mindfulness for Smoking Cessation: A Guide to Controlling Your Craving Using Mindfulness-Based Strategies" by Shahroo Izadi:

Mindfulness-based strategies have been proven effective in various areas of personal development, including smoking cessation. This book provides pregnant women with practical tools and exercises to manage cravings, cope with stress, and shift their mindset towards quitting. By incorporating mindfulness into our daily lives, we can create new habits and decrease dependency on smoking while simultaneously creating a nurturing environment for our babies.

Healthcare Providers and Counselling Services

Finding the Right Healthcare Professionals:

Choosing the right healthcare provider is essential, as they will be your partner throughout your pregnancy journey. When it comes to quitting smoking, it is crucial to find a healthcare provider who has experience in smoking cessation programs and is well-informed about the risks associated with smoking during pregnancy.

To find the right healthcare provider, you can start by seeking recommendations from friends, family, or your primary care physician. You can also utilize online resources and review websites to get a sense of the experiences other pregnant women have had with various healthcare providers.

Once you have a shortlist of potential healthcare providers, schedule an initial consultation to discuss your pregnancy and your desire to quit smoking. Use this opportunity to ask questions, gauge their knowledge and experience in smoking cessation, and assess their communication style. It is vital to have a healthcare provider who not only possesses the necessary expertise but also connects with you on a personal level, making you feel comfortable and supported throughout your journey.

Scheduling Appointments:

Regular consultations with your healthcare provider are crucial during pregnancy, especially when you are trying to quit smoking. These appointments serve as an opportunity for your provider to monitor your progress and address any concerns or challenges you may be facing.

When scheduling appointments, make sure to prioritize your health and well-being. Find a healthcare provider who offers convenient appointment times that align with your schedule. It is also important to consider factors such as the location of the healthcare facility, the availability of transportation options, and any other logistical considerations that may impact your ability to attend appointments regularly.

Utilizing Counselling Services:

In addition to healthcare providers, counselling services can offer pregnant women invaluable support during the journey to quit smoking. Counselling services provide a non-judgmental space for pregnant women to explore their smoking habits, understand the underlying reasons for their addiction, and develop strategies to overcome cravings and withdrawal symptoms.

There are several types of counselling services available, and it is important to choose the one that aligns with your needs and preferences. One-on-one counselling sessions with a licensed counsellor or therapist offer personalized support and guidance tailored to your specific circumstances. Group counselling sessions, on the other hand, provide an opportunity to connect with other pregnant women facing similar challenges and share experiences and strategies for success.

When seeking counselling services, it is crucial to ensure that the counsellors or therapists have experience in working with pregnant women and smoking cessation. Ask for references or recommendations from healthcare providers or other trusted sources to ensure that you are receiving the most effective and appropriate support.

It is worth noting that counselling services can be offered in various formats, including in-person, over the phone, or through online platforms. Choose the format that suits your preferences and circumstances, considering factors such as accessibility, convenience, and comfort.

Remember, quitting smoking is a journey, and it is okay to seek support. Your healthcare providers and counselling services are there to guide and assist you every step of the way. With dedication, perseverance, and the assistance of these professionals, you can empower yourself to quit smoking and provide the best possible start for your baby's life.

Remember, your story is powerful and has the potential to impact the lives of others. By sharing your journey, you are not only celebrating your own success but also contributing to a larger movement of empowering and inspiring pregnant women to choose a smoke-free life.

In conclusion, celebrating the journey of pregnant women who have successfully quit smoking is vital for inspiring others and fostering a sense of community and support. By sharing our stories, we show others that they are not alone and that there is hope for a smoke-free future. Celebrating personal achievements boosts self-esteem and self-worth while creating a safe and nurturing environment for everyone involved. I encourage all pregnant women

who have quit smoking to share their success stories
and be part of a movement that empowers and
inspires others on their journey to a smoke-free life.

www.ingramcontent.com/pod-product-compliance
Lightning Source LLC
Chambersburg PA
CBHW070837260726

48660CB00005B/2075